Molecular
Medicine

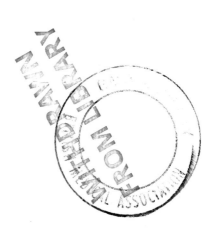

Molecular Medicine

JOHN BRADLEY

BMedSci, MA, DM, FRCP
University of Cambridge School of Clinical Medicine
Addenbrooke's Hospital, Cambridge, UK

DAVID JOHNSON

PhD
Department of Pathology
Yale Medical School
New Haven, Connecticut, USA

DAVID RUBENSTEIN

MA, MD, FRCP (Lond)
University of Cambridge School of Clinical Medicine
Addenbrooke's Hospital, Cambridge, UK

Second Edition

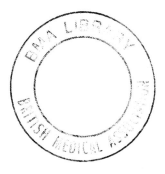

Blackwell
Science

A catalogue record for this title
is available from the British Library

ISBN 0-632-05839-0

Library of Congress
Cataloging-in-Publication Data
Bradley, John, MRCP.
 Lecture notes on molecular
medicine /
 John Bradley, David Johnson, David
Rubenstein.—2nd ed.
   p. ;   cm.
 Includes index.
 ISBN 0-632-05839-0 (pbk.)
 1. Molecular biology—Outlines,
syllabi, etc.
 2. Molecular genetics—Outlines,
syllabi, etc.
 3. Medical genetics—Outlines, syllabi,
etc.
 4. Pathology, Molecular—Outlines,
syllabi, etc.
 I. Title: Molecular medicine.
 II. Johnson, David, Ph. D.
 III. Rubenstein, David.   IV. Title.
   [DNLM: 1. Genetics,
Biochemical—Outlines.
 2. Genetic Techniques—Outlines.
 QU 18.2 B811m 2001]
 QH506 .B734 2001
 616'.042—dc21
                    2001025377

DISTRIBUTORS

 Marston Book Services Ltd
 PO Box 269
 Abingdon, Oxon OX14 4YN
 (Orders: Tel: 01235 465500
      Fax: 01235 465555)

The Americas
 Blackwell Publishing
 c/o AIDC
 PO Box 20
 50 Winter Sport Lane
 Williston, VT 05495-0020
 (Orders: Tel: 800 216 2522
      Fax: 802 864 7626)

Australia
 Blackwell Science Pty Ltd
 54 University Street
 Carlton, Victoria 3053
 (Orders: Tel: 3 9347 0300
      Fax: 3 9347 5001)

For further information on
Blackwell Science, visit our website:
www.blackwell-science.com

Contents

Preface

To the second edition

The text has been updated to include recent advances, particularly where related to clinical disease. We are particularly grateful for the many complimentary comments and constructive suggestions received, many of which have now been incorporated. It has been most encouraging to discover the numbers successfully using the book as a primer for what, on first encounter, appears a difficult and daunting subject. We hope that we have dispelled that belief.

Blackwell Science, as ever, remain wonderfully supportive.

To the first edition

Molecular medicine is a novel, exciting and important subject which is made difficult by an unfamiliar language. In the first part of this book we have attempted to introduce the discipline to the new reader, using an extensively illustrated text to explain the common terms and their applications. The second part of the book outlines how molecular biology is used to define the molecular basis of disease. Finally, we describe how this is beginning to translate into benefits for patients.

We would like to thank Kathleen Gillespie, Richard Sandford and Phil Roberts for reading the text. We are particularly grateful to Jordan Pober for his comments and advice. Brad Amos generously gave his expert help in preparing the confocal micrographs for the cover and chapter headings.

Abbreviations

A	adenine		eNOS	endothelial nitric oxide synthase
ACE	angiotensin-converting enzyme		ES	embryonic stem
ACTH	adrenocorticotrophic hormone		EST	expressed sequence tag
AD	transcription-activating domain		EtBr	ethidium bromide
ADA	adenosine deaminase		FISH	fluorescent *in situ* hybridization
AFP	α-fetoprotein		FRET	fluorescence resonance energy
ApoE	apolipoprotein E			transfer
APP	β-amyloid precursor protein		G	guanine
ARMS	amplification refractory mutation		GFP	green fluorescent protein
	system		GM-CSF	granulocyte–macrophage colony-
AZT	azidothymidine			stimulating factor
BAC	bacterial artificial chromosome		GST	glutathione-S-transferase
BLAST	basic local alignment search tool		HA	haemagglutinin
bp	base pair(s)		hCG	human chorionic gonadotrophin
B/Y/CFP	blue/yellow/cyan fluorescent		HERVs	human endogenous retroviruses
	protein		hGH	human growth hormone
C	cytosine		HGP	Human Genome Project
CAT	chloramphenicol acetyl transferase		HGPRT	hypoxanthine guanine
cDNA	complementary DNA			phosphoribosyl transferase
CFTR	cystic fibrosis transmembrane		HIV	human immunodeficiency virus
	conductance regulator		HLA	human leucocyte antigen
CGH	comparative genomic		hnRNA	heterogeneous nuclear RNA
	hybridization		HSV-1	herpes simplex virus type 1
CNS	central nervous system		HTF	*Hpa*II tiny fragments
CTLs	cytotoxic T lymphocytes		HUGO	Human Genome Organization
DAF	decay accelerating factor		ICAM	intercellular adhesion molecule
DBD	DNA-binding domain		IDDM	insulin-dependent diabetes
ddI	didanosine			mellitus
ddNTP	dideoxynucleotide		IEF	isoelectric focusing
DEPC	diethylpyrocarbonate		IGF	insulin-like growth factor
DHFR	dihydrofolate reductase		IL	interleukin
DMS	dimethylsulphate		IVS	intervening sequence
DNA	deoxyribonucleic acid		LDL	low density lipoprotein
dNTP	deoxynucleotide		LFA	leucocyte function-associated
EDTA	ethylene diamine tetra-acetic acid			antigen
eIF	elongation factor		LOD	logarithm of the odds
EMSA	electrophoretic mobility shift		LTR	long terminal repeat
	assay		MCP	membrane cofactor protein

MEN	multiple endocrine neoplasia	RNasin	RNase inhibitor
MHC	major histocompatibility complex	rNTP	ribonucleotide
MODY	maturity-onset diabetes of the young	rRNA	ribosomal RNA
		RT	reverse transcriptase
mRNA	messenger RNA	SAGE	serial analysis of gene expression
MSC	Mouse Sequencing Consortium	SCID	severe combined immunodeficiency
NASBA	nucleic acid synthesis-based amplification	SDS	sodium dodecyl sulphate
NIDDM	non-insulin-dependent diabetes mellitus	SNP	single nucleotide polymorphism
		SNuPE	single nucleotide primer extension
NIH	National Institute of Health	SSCP	single-strand conformation polymorphism
NO	nitric oxide		
OD	optical density	STS	sequence-tagged site
PCR	polymerase chain reaction	T	thymine
PDGF	platelet-derived growth factor	TAR	trans-activation response region
PEG	polyethylene glycol	TdT	terminal deoxytransferase
PFGE	pulsed field gel electrophoresis	TFO	triplex-forming oligonucleotide
PNA	peptide nucleic acid	t-PA	tissue-type plasminogen activator
Pol	polymerase	tRNA	transfer RNA
RAC	Recombinant DNA Advisory Committee	U	uracil
RAPD	randomly amplified polymorphic DNA	UTR	untranslated region
		UV	ultraviolet
RBC	red blood cell	VEGF	vascular endothelial cell growth factor
RCA	rolling circle amplification		
RFLP	restriction fragment length polymorphism	VNTR	variable number of tandem repeats
rhDNase	recombinant human deoxyribonuclease	WASP	Wiskott–Aldrich syndrome protein
RNA	ribonucleic acid	XIST	X-inactivation-specific transcript
RNase	ribonuclease	YAC	yeast artificial chromosome

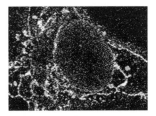

Basic Principles

Molecular biology is a fascinating subject.

Viruses and prokaryotic organisms ensure their survival by using a variety of techniques to make, break and join DNA.

Viruses are small cellular parasites that generally consist of DNA or ribonucleic acid (RNA) with a protein coat. In some complex viruses a membrane surrounds the protein coat.

Prokaryotic organism—simple, single-cell life form that lacks a distinct nucleus. Examples include bacteria and certain algae.

The adoption of these techniques by molecular biologists has led to remarkable breakthroughs in molecular biology in recent decades.

In this chapter we will describe in detail how information is stored in DNA, and how this information is used by the cell.

Organisms are made of cells

Living organisms are composed of cells. Some organisms, including bacteria, algae and yeasts, exist as single cells, whereas plants and animals consist of collections of cells. New cells, required for growth of an existing organism or the formation of new organisms, arise by division of existing cells.

Cell functions depend on proteins

All cellular functions depend on proteins, which consist of chains of amino acids. Only 20 different amino acids are commonly found in the proteins of all organisms.

The links in a chain of amino acids are termed peptide bonds, and the chains themselves are called polypeptides. Proteins contain one or more polypeptides, and the structure and function of each protein depends on the sequence of amino acids making up the polypeptide chains.

Proteins have many diverse functions. They maintain cell structure and provide motility, act as intra- and extracellular messengers, and bind and transport molecules, including oxygen, lipids and other proteins. Many proteins are enzymes which catalyse (accelerate) chemical reactions. Almost all chemical reactions, including those involved in the synthesis of fats and carbohydrates, are catalysed by enzymes.

Some proteins, e.g. the enzymes involved in glucose metabolism, occur in most cells. In contrast, cells in multicellular organisms may become specialized and produce certain proteins that provide them with highly specific functions. Cells that produce particular proteins are often grouped together to form complex tissues or organs. For example, muscle cells produce proteins, including tropomyosin and myosin, which are involved in the formation of muscle filaments, islet cells of the pancreas synthesize the polypeptide hormone insulin, and

1

liver cells contain enzymes found exclusively in the liver, such as those required for the conjugation of bilirubin into water-soluble forms.

> In RNA the sugar is ribose, uracil replaces T and the resulting nucleic acid is single stranded.

DNA contains the information needed to encode proteins

Cells therefore need:
• the information to produce proteins in a regulated fashion; and
• the ability to convey this information to daughter cells during cell division.

The key to these requirements is provided by the DNA *double helix*, which contains two strands of DNA held together by weak chemical interactions.

The strands complement each other—the sequences of bases on one strand can be determined from the sequence of the other strand. During cell division each strand independently forms a new complementary strand, and the DNA helix is able to direct its own duplication.

BASIC DNA STRUCTURE

Each strand of DNA has a backbone of sugars and phosphates, with a nitrogen-containing base attached to each sugar. Four different bases are found in DNA. Cytosine (C) and thymine (T) are pyrimidines which contain one nitrogenous ring, whereas adenine (A) and guanine (G) are purines which contain two. The bases from each strand are linked together to form the 'rungs' inside the helix in such a way that A can only pair with T, and C can only pair with G.

The sequence of bases in a DNA molecule carries the information that specifies the order of amino acids along a polypeptide chain. Each of the 20 amino acids is encoded by coding units, or codons, which consist of three consecutive bases. Reading this code, and translating it into protein, requires ribonucleic acid (RNA).

A segment of DNA that carries the information needed to encode a specific polypeptide is known as a gene. To retrieve this information a single-stranded messenger RNA (mRNA) copy of the gene is made, and the sequence of bases in the mRNA is then translated into a linear sequence of amino acids, composing a polypeptide. Genetic information is therefore stored in cells in DNA. During the expression of a gene, a segment of DNA is first transcribed into RNA, and then translated from RNA into protein. During cell division DNA replicates itself to form two identical DNA helices.

DNA in eukaryotic organisms is organized into chromosomes within the cell nucleus

Living things may be divided into prokaryotes and eukaryotes. Prokaryotic organisms are simple, single-cell life forms that lack a distinct nucleus. Examples include bacteria and certain algae. The cells in eukaryotic organisms contain nuclei. Eukaryotes may be single-cell life forms such as yeasts, or complex multicellular organisms such as plants and animals. DNA within the nucleus of eukaryotes is organized into chromosomes. Each chromosome contains an extensively folded, DNA double helix.

DNA

DNA is composed of three principal structures:
• bases;
• sugars;
• phosphates.
These are kept together by three principal types of linkage:
• covalent bond;
• hydrogen bond;
• ester link.

The players

Bases

The bases in DNA are nitrogen-containing rings (the nitrogen makes these molecules basic). Pyrimidines (C, T) have one ring, whilst purines (A, G) have two.

> Base—a molecule that can combine with hydrogen ions in solution.

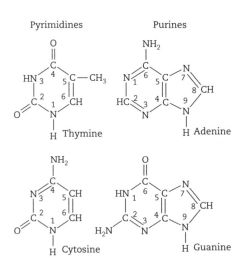

Pyrimidines   Purines

Thymine   Adenine

Cytosine   Guanine

Sugars

The sugars in DNA are pentoses (sugar molecules containing five carbon atoms). In DNA the pentose is always deoxyribose, indicating that it lacks an oxygen molecule that is present in ribose, the parent compound.

> Ribose could not fit into a DNA helix as there is insufficient room for the 2'-OH group.

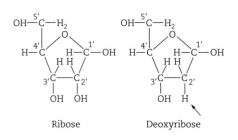

Ribose   Deoxyribose

By convention the carbon atoms are labelled by primed numbers (1' to 5') when part of a nucleotide. This labelling is important in understanding how the DNA molecule is assembled.

Phosphates

The phosphates in DNA are either mono-, di- or triphosphates. The acidic character of nucleic acid is due to the presence of phosphate esters, which are relatively strong acids.

> Acid—a molecule that releases a hydrogen ion in solution.

At neutral pH they dissociate from hydrogen ions, and are thus normally referred to in their ionized form:

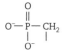 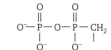

Monophosphonate   Diphosphonate

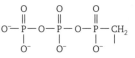

Triphosphonate

The ties that bind

Covalent bonds

> A covalent bond exists between atoms that share electrons in their outermost shell. The bonding electrons move freely around both nuclei which are held close together in a strong bond—energy is released when the bonds are formed, and the same amount of energy is required to break the bond.

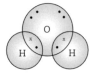

In water each hydrogen atom shares its electron (x) with an electron from the outer shell of the oxygen atom (•). The hydrogen atom thus fills its outer (first) shell with two electrons, and the oxygen atom fills its outer (second) shell with eight

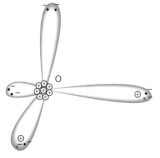

Outer orbitals have characteristic shapes. The four outer orbitals of an oxygen atom in water point outwards, forming the corners of a tetrahedron

Hydrogen bond

A hydrogen atom can usually only form one covalent bond with another atom. A covalently bonded (*electron-depleted*) hydrogen atom can, however, form a weak electrostatic inter-action (*hydrogen bond*) with an electronegative (*electron-rich*) atom (usually nitrogen or oxygen), e.g.

N —— H --- O

Covalent   Hydrogen
bond   bond

Ester linkage

An ester link involves covalent bonding. It is formed when an alcohol and an acid unite with elimination of water.

BOND STRENGTH

The strength of the bonds is important in understanding the stability of different parts of the final DNA molecule. Strong covalent bonds link nucleic acids in a single DNA strand, whereas weaker hydrogen bonds hold two DNA strands together.

The formation of DNA

Base + sugar = nucleoside

The 1′ carbon of pentose ring is attached to nitrogen 1 of pyrimidine or nitrogen 9 of purine.

Nitrogen 1 of pyrimidine   Nitrogen 9 of purine
(e.g. thymine)   (e.g. guanine)

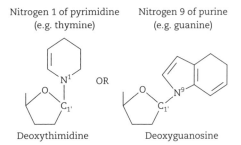

OR

Deoxythimidine   Deoxyguanosine

Base + sugar + phosphate = nucleotide

Phosphate is attached to the 5′-carbon of the pentose ring.

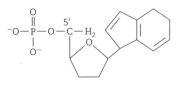

Deoxyguanosine 5'-phosphate

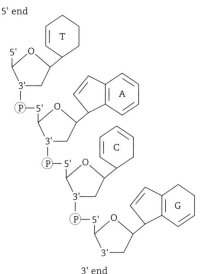

5' end

3' end

NUCLEOTIDES AS ENERGY STORES

Nucleotides may have either one, two or three phosphates attached. In addition to forming the building blocks of DNA, the nucleotide di- and triphosphates are important stores of chemical energy; cleavage of the terminal phosphate bond releases energy which is used to drive cell functions. Adenosine triphosphate (ATP) is the most widely used energy carrier in the cell.

Nucleotides join together to form nucleic acid

The hydroxyl group attached to the 3'-pentose carbon of one nucleotide forms an ester link with the phosphate of another molecule, eliminating a water molecule. The link between nucleotides is known as a phosphodiester link.

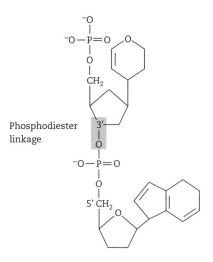

Phosphodiester linkage

Thus, one end of a DNA strand has a sugar residue in which the 5'-carbon is not linked to another sugar residue (the 5' end), whereas at the other end the 3'-carbon lacks a phosphodiester link (the 3' end).

This simple terminology is fundamental to understanding descriptions of how DNA replicates and is expressed.

DNA structure

The DNA helix

In the 1950s X-ray diffraction data suggested that DNA is helical (Fig. 1.1a). In addition, biochemical data showed that the amount of A in DNA always equalled that of T, whilst the amount of G equalled that of C. These observations led Watson and Crick to propose the double helical structure of DNA, which could account for the physical properties of DNA and its replication in the cell.

The 'backbone' on the outside of the helix consists of alternating sugars and phosphates. The bases are attached to the sugars and form the 'rungs' of the helix.

As the distance between the sugar–phosphate backbone is fixed by the diameter of helix, only two types of base pairs (AT or CG) can fit, explaining the constant regularity in the ratios between base pairs (A = T and G = C) (Fig. 1.1c).

The strands are antiparallel (their 5',3'-phosphodiester links run in opposite directions) and complementary (because of base pairing the chains complement each other). The sequences

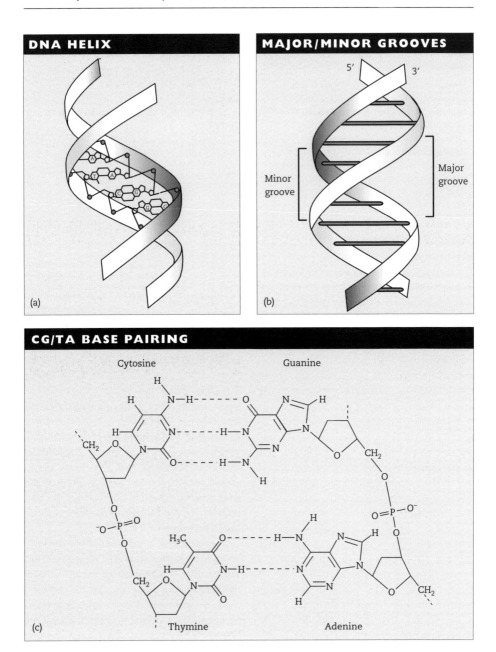

DNA HELIX

(a)

MAJOR/MINOR GROOVES

5′   3′

Minor groove

Major groove

(b)

CG/TA BASE PAIRING

Cytosine   Guanine

Thymine   Adenine

(c)

Fig. 1.1 (a) Diagrammatic representation of the DNA helix. (b) The major and minor grooves of the DNA helix. (c) CG/TA base pairing.

of bases on one strand can thus be deduced from the sequences of bases on the other, and each strand independently carries the information needed to form a double helix.

The DNA helix can take on several conformations. The most common form is *B-DNA*,

CLEAVAGE OF DNA BONDS

The relative weakness of the hydrogen bonds holding the base pairs together is demonstrated by 'melting' the DNA. At increased temperatures the two strands separate: the DNA melts.

The bonds holding the backbone of the helix together are stronger and do not melt, but can be cleaved by enzymes derived from bacteria which cut the backbone at specific sites.

Bacteria use these enzymes as protective devices to degrade foreign DNA. They restrict the growth of viruses which infect bacteria (bacteriophages), and are known as restriction enzymes.

A bacteriophage is a virus that infects bacteria, sometimes referred to as a phage.

DESCRIBING A DNA SEQUENCE

It is conventional to describe a DNA sequence by writing the sequence of bases in one strand only, and in the 5′ → 3′ direction. When identifying just two neighbouring bases in a sequence it is usual to insert 'p' between them to denote an intervening phosphodiester link (e.g. ApT). This is distinct from AT which indicates a hydrogen-bonded base pair on complementary strands.

in which the helix is right-handed and has just over 10 base pairs (bp) per helical turn. There are two unequal grooves, the major and minor grooves (Fig. 1.1b).

A-DNA is a right-handed helix which is shorter and wider than B-DNA. The phosphate groups bind fewer water molecules, and its formation is thus favoured by dehydration.

Z-DNA is a left-handed helix in which alternating purines and pyrimidines give rise to a zigzag appearance to the helix.

Chromatin

The total length of all the strands of DNA in a human cell is ~2 m, all of which needs to be packed into a nucleus a few micrometres in diameter. This is achieved by the formation of a nucleoprotein complex called *chromatin*: acidic phosphates in the backbone of DNA enable it to form ionic bonds with basic lysine- and arginine-rich proteins known as histones. Coiling of DNA around histone proteins allows long strands to be tightly packed into chromatin.

DNA is first packaged into a *nucleosome* (Fig. 1.2), which consists of eight histone proteins around which a strand of DNA containing 146 bp is wound one and three-quarter times.

NUCLEOSOME

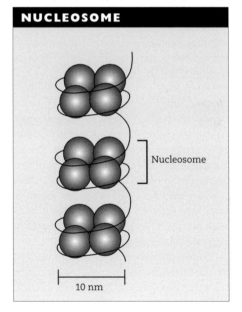

Fig. 1.2 A nucleosome.

There are five major histone proteins termed H1, H2A, H2B, H3 and H4. The core of the nucleosome contains two copies each of H2A, H2B, H3 and H4.

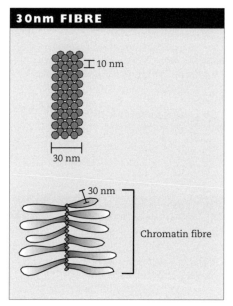

Fig. 1.3 A chromatin 30 nm fibre.

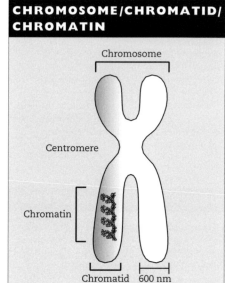

Fig. 1.4 Chromosomes, chromatids and chromatin.

The histone protein H1 binds to DNA just next to each nucleosome, and is involved in coiling DNA into chromatin fibres of 30 nm in diameter (Fig. 1.3).

Chromosomes

During cell division chromatin becomes more condensed, and can be recognized in the form of *chromosomes* by light microscopy. During metaphase each chromosome consists of two symmetrical *chromatids*, each containing DNA in which the chromatin fibres are folded in loops around a central scaffold of non-histone acidic protein. The chromatids are attached to each other at the centromere (Fig. 1.4).

Condensed metaphase chromosomes can be subdivided by various treatments which cause the appearance of light and dark bands. For example, staining with Giemsa gives rise to alternating dark- and pale-staining *G bands* (Fig. 1.5). Such banding allows classification of sites on the chromosome according to their location on the short arm (p for petit), or long arm (q), and their position relative to the centromere. For example, the gene that encodes the β-globin chain of haemoglobin (which is

DNA IN PROKARYOTES

In prokaryotes all the DNA exists in a single molecule which is circular. There are no 5′ or 3′ ends and no histones, and there is no nucleus. The DNA can, however, be induced to supercoil into a compact structure around DNA-binding proteins by the enzyme DNA gyrase.

abnormal in β thalassaemia), has been localized to the short arm of chromosome 11, in region 1, band 5, sub-band 5: written as 11p15.5 (Fig. 1.5).

Karyotype

Every species has a specific number and form of chromosomes, which is referred to as a *karyotype*. Human cells contain 46 chromosomes, of which two are sex chromosomes (two X chromosomes in females, an X and a Y chromosome in males), and 44 are autosomes (22 matching pairs numbered 1–22) (Fig. 1.6).

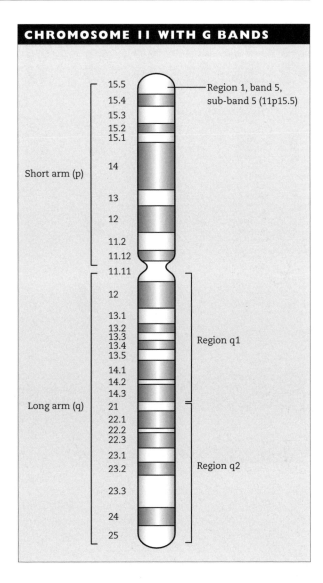

CHROMOSOME 11 WITH G BANDS

Region 1, band 5, sub-band 5 (11p15.5)

Short arm (p)

15.5
15.4
15.3
15.2
15.1

14

13

12

11.2
11.12
11.11

12

13.1
13.2
13.3
13.4
13.5

14.1
14.2
14.3
21
22.1
22.2
22.3

23.1
23.2

23.3

24

25

Long arm (q)

Region q1

Region q2

Fig. 1.5 Chromosome 11 with G bands.

Genome

The complete genetic make-up of an individual is referred to as their *genome*. Thus, in human cells the genome is composed of 23 pairs of chromosomes within the nucleus, each chromosome containing a single, linear, double helical strand of DNA. The human genome contains approximately 3×10^9 bp (base pairs), and is thought to contain about 30 000 different genes, most of which encode polypeptides. A small minority of genes encode RNA molecules.

In addition to the nuclear genome, eukaryotic cells also contain a small mitochondrial genome which tends to be inherited from the mother. This is because, unlike sperm, eggs have a considerable amount of cytoplasm which contains mitochondria. In humans the mitochondrial genome consists of a 16 569-bp circular DNA molecule which encodes proteins essential for mitochondrial structure and function, including oxidative enzymes, together with RNA molecules involved in mitochondrial protein synthesis.

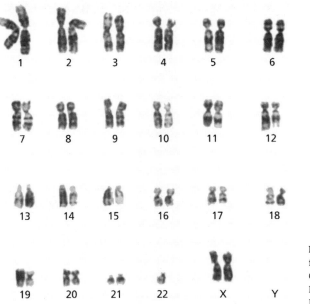

Fig. 1.6 A normal human female karyotype stained with Giemsa. Courtesy of Genetics Laboratories, Addenbrooke's Hospital, Cambridge.

Although mitochondria possess their own genome, the majority of mitochondrial proteins are encoded by nuclear genes.

The code carried by mRNA is read and translated into protein in ribosomes. Ribosomes are structures found in the cytoplasm of cells, composed of ribosomal RNA (rRNA) and ribosomal proteins.

RNA structure

DNA carries the information that encodes polypeptides. Reading this code, and translating it into specific proteins, involves RNA.

RNA differs from DNA in the following respects:
• RNA is single stranded (usually);
• the sugar in RNA is ribose rather than deoxyribose;
• RNA has uracil (U) rather than T as one of its pyrimidines.

RNA exists in three forms.
• *Messenger RNA (mRNA)* is a copy of DNA which encodes a specific amino acid sequence.
• *Transfer RNA (tRNA)* carries amino acids to ribosomes.
• *Ribosomal RNA (rRNA)* facilitates the interaction between mRNA and tRNA, resulting in the translation of mRNA into protein.

Whilst mRNA is formed as a copy of a gene encoding a specific polypeptide, tRNA and rRNA are formed as the products of genes which actually encode RNA molecules. Multiple copies of genes encoding different tRNA and rRNA molecules occur.

DNA replication and transcription: it's all in the genes

The double helical structure of DNA provides a mechanism by which nucleic acids can accurately replicate and provide the information for building proteins.

During replication the two chains dissociate and each one serves as a template for the synthesis of two complementary strands of

tRNA AND rRNA

tRNA molecules differ according to the amino acid they carry. About 1600 copies of genes encoding different tRNA molecules are dispersed throughout the human genome.

rRNA is formed of different-sized subunits, designated 28S, 5.8S, 18S and 5S. The 28S, 5.8S and 18S subunits are formed by processing a large precursor RNA molecule encoded by about 300 copies of a gene which occurs on chromosomes 13, 14, 15, 21 and 22. Copies of the gene encoding the 5S subunit are clustered together on chromosome 1.

Subunits of RNA are commonly designated S, or Svedberg units, which are related to the size and shape of the RNA. Svedberg units are actually measures of the sedimentation rate of molecules centrifuged through a density gradient. This was a common method of analysing macromolecules before gel electrophoresis (see p. 32) became routine.

DNA. During gene expression information is retrieved from only one of the two available strands. The segment of DNA containing a gene is first transcribed into a single-stranded mRNA copy which has the same sequence of bases as the sense strand of DNA, and is complementary to the antisense strand. The sequence of bases is then translated into a sequence of amino acids composing a polypeptide (see p. 23).

> The sense strand of DNA has the same sequence of bases as the transcribed mRNA (in which U replaces T). The antisense strand carries the complementary sequence of bases.

> The direction of synthesis of DNA during replication, or RNA during transcription, is $5' \rightarrow 3'$.

The flow of genetic information in a cell can thus be summarized as follows.

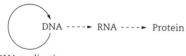

DNA replication

When viruses are taken into consideration, genetic information can also pass from RNA to RNA during replication of some RNA viruses, and from RNA to DNA in retroviruses, which

VIRUSES

Viruses are small cellular parasites which generally consist of DNA or RNA within a protein coat or capsid. In some complex viruses a membrane surrounds the protein coat. A virus cannot replicate by itself, but uses the machinery of infected cells to do so.

have RNA genomes from which a DNA copy is made during their infectious cycle. The retrovirus genome contains the gene for the enzyme reverse transcriptase which catalyses RNA-dependent synthesis of DNA.

DNA replication

For DNA replication to occur the following are required.

• A DNA *template* containing a region of single-stranded DNA from which a complementary copy is made. The double-stranded helix must unwind, and each strand then acts as a template. DNA helicase stimulates separation of the two strands. DNA gyrase aids unwinding by catalysing formation of negative supercoils (see p. 35) and DNA single-stranded binding proteins stabilize the single-stranded structure.

> DNA replication is *semiconservative*—one strand (half of the original DNA) is retained ('conserved') in the new DNA molecule.

• A *primer* chain with a free 3'-OH group at the site where replication originates.

The primer is a short strand of RNA which is synthesized on the template at the start of replication, and removed at the end—RNA *primes the synthesis of* DNA.

• A supply of *triphosphate nucleosides* to attach to the growing chain.
• *DNA polymerases* (Pols) which catalyse the addition of nucleotides to the pre-existing strand of DNA or primer RNA.

DNA Pols produce a link between the inner phosphorus of the nucleotide and the 3'-OH group of the primer—elongation occurs in the $5' \rightarrow 3'$ direction.

• The whole process requires *energy* which is supplied by the hydrolysis of nucleoside triphosphates releasing pyrophosphate. The enzyme pyrophosphatase splits the high-energy phosphoanhydride bond in pyrophosphate, which is converted to inorganic phosphate.

Much of our understanding of how DNA replicates (Fig. 1.7) has come from the study of the bacterium *Escherichia coli*, in which DNA is present as a single circular molecule. Replication starts at a specific site (the site of origin, *oriC*), and proceeds sequentially in opposite directions, even though synthesis can only occur in the $5' \rightarrow 3'$ direction. This apparent paradox was resolved by the demonstration that synthesis of one strand occurs continuously, whereas the other strand is synthesized in short $5'–3'$ fragments (Okazaki fragments), which are then joined together by DNA ligase.

E. coli actually contains three different DNA Pols (I, II and III) which catalyse both the formation and hydrolysis of DNA. The first DNA Pol to be described, DNA Pol I, was found to have three different enzymatic activities:
• a polymerase that catalyses the formation of new phosphodiester bonds in the growing DNA chain;

• a $3'–5'$ exonuclease that catalyses the removal of nucleotides from the 3' end of DNA chains;

The $3'–5'$ exonuclease is thought to edit each newly attached base, and remove any which are mismatched and will not fit into a double helix.

• a $5'–3'$ exonuclease that cleaves bonds within one chain of a double helix.

$5'–3'$ exonucleases remove the RNA primer and are thought to repair double-stranded DNA that is damaged.

Polymerase I can itself be cleaved to yield two fragments: a small fragment containing the $5'–3'$ exonuclease, and a large fragment (the Klenow fragment) with DNA polymerase and $3'–5'$ exonuclease activity:

Klenow fragment

N-----------C N----------------------C
5'-3' exonuclease   3'-5' exonuclease polymerase

Small fragment   Large fragment
                     (Klenow fragment)

The Klenow fragment is used by molecular biologists to accurately synthesize DNA strands.

Most of the DNA in *E. coli* is in fact synthesized by Pol III, whereas repair of the DNA and removal of the RNA primer is predominantly performed by Pol I.

A similar mechanism for DNA replication occurs in eukaryotic cells, although the process differs in the following respects.
• Polymerases in eukaryotic cells include polymerase α, β, δ (located in the nucleus) and γ (located in mitochondria).
• Because of the size of eukaryotic genomes, replication originates at many sites within each chromosome.

DNA REPLICATION

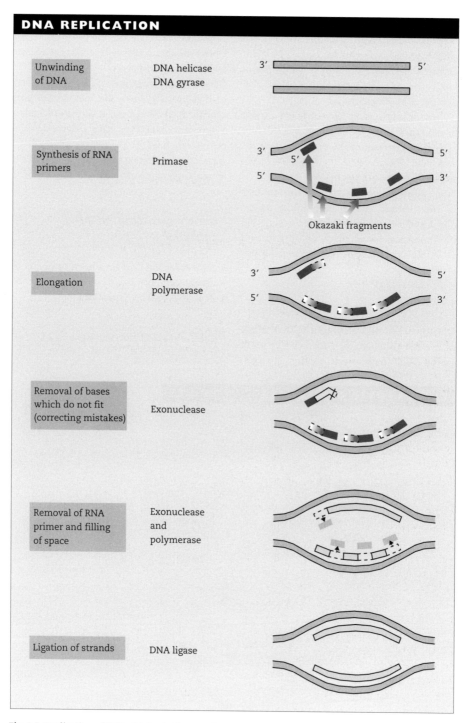

Unwinding of DNA	DNA helicase DNA gyrase	
Synthesis of RNA primers	Primase	Okazaki fragments
Elongation	DNA polymerase	
Removal of bases which do not fit (correcting mistakes)	Exonuclease	
Removal of RNA primer and filling of space	Exonuclease and polymerase	
Ligation of strands	DNA ligase	

Fig. 1.7 Replication of DNA: driving both ways down a one-way street.

• DNA replication is a virtually continuous process in prokaryotic cells—as soon as the chromosome has duplicated, the two daughter chromosomes segregate and the cell divides. In eukaryotic cells DNA synthesis and cell division occur at different times.

The whole process of cell growth and division in eukaryotic cells can be divided into different phases, which together make up the cell cycle.

Eukaryotic cell cycle

The eukaryotic cell cycle (Fig. 1.8) consists of two periods: (i) the M (mitotic) period (Fig. 1.9) during which cell division occurs; and (ii) interphase during which cell growth and DNA replication occur. Interphase is further divided into:
• G1 (gap 1);
• S (synthetic);
• G2 (gap 2) phases.
DNA synthesis occurs only during the S phase of the cell cycle, which is followed by a gap period (G2) before cell division (mitosis)

occurs. Mitosis is followed by a further gap period (G1) during which the cell prepares for DNA synthesis. Cells which are not preparing for DNA synthesis and cell division may leave G1 and enter a stage called G0. Such cells may be metabolically active, but they do not proceed through the cell cycle. G0 may represent a temporary quiescent state, from which the cell returns to G1, or a terminally differentiated state. Non-replicating cells such as nerve cells are generally stopped in G0.

Gene expression: making proteins

Gene expression involves the transcription of a segment of DNA into RNA, and the translation of RNA into a polypeptide.

> A *gene* is a sequence of DNA which codes for one polypeptide.

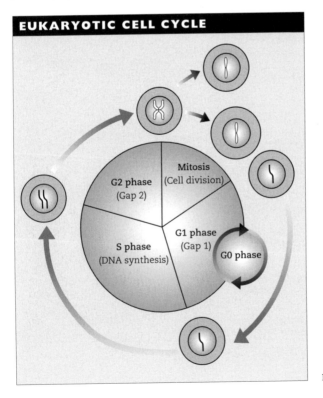

EUKARYOTIC CELL CYCLE

G2 phase (Gap 2)

Mitosis (Cell division)

S phase (DNA synthesis)

G1 phase (Gap 1)

G0 phase

Fig. 1.8 Eukaryotic cell cycle.

MITOSIS

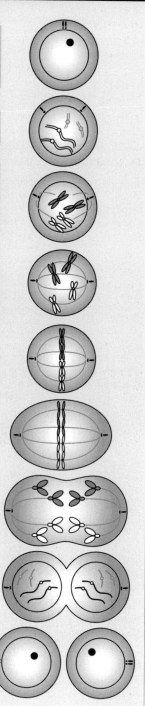

Interphase Replication of DNA occurs, but chromosomes are not distinguishable by light microscopy. DNA involved in synthesis of RNA is condensed into the nucleolus. The two centrioles duplicate to form daughters

Early prophase The chromosomes appear as long threads. The nucleolus disperses and the centrioles start separating

Middle prophase Chromosomes condense to form chromatids, each containing one of the two DNA molecules that were produced during interphase. The centrioles, which are constructed of microtubules, start to form a spindle as they move to opposite poles of the cell

Late prophase The centrioles reach the poles and are linked by spindle fibres that extend to the centre (equator) of the cell, or attach to the kinetochore (close to the centromere) of each chromatid. The nuclear membrane disperses and disappears

Metaphase The chromatids become aligned on the equator

Early anaphase The two chromatids separate

Late anaphase Each set of chromatids (now a new set of chromosomes) moves to each pole. Separation of the cell cytoplasm (cytokinesis) begins

Telophase Nuclear membranes form around the separated chromosomes, which uncoil and become less distinct. Cytokinesis continues and the spindle disappears

Interphase Following completion of cell division, DNA replication starts again

Fig. 1.9 Mitosis.

GENETIC CODING

Each of the 20 amino acids (for abbreviations see below) is encoded by a triplet of bases (*codon*). Since there are four bases there are $4 \times 4 \times 4 = 64$ possible codons, and single amino acids may be encoded by more than one codon (there is 'redundancy' in the code).

Certain codons specify the beginning and end of polypeptide chains. Methionine, encoded by AUG (or more rarely GAG, which usually encodes valine), is found at the start of polypeptide chains, whereas UAA, UAG and UGA do not specify amino acids, but indicate termination or stop signals at the end of chains.

POSSIBLE CODONS OF AN AMINO ACID

First position (5′ end)	Second position				Third position (3′ end)
	U	C	A	G	
U	Phe (UUU)	Ser (UCU)	Tyr (UAU)	Cys (UGU)	U
	Phe (UUC)	Ser (UCC)	Tyr (UAC)	Cys (UGC)	C
	Leu (UUA)	Ser (UCA)	Stop (UAA)	Stop (UGA)	A
	Leu (UUG)	Ser (UCG)	Stop (UAG)	Trp (UGG)	G
C	Leu (CUU)	Pro (CCU)	His (CAU)	Arg (CGU)	U
	Leu (CUC)	Pro (CCC)	His (CAC)	Arg (CGC)	C
	Leu (CUA)	Pro (CCA)	Gln (CAA)	Arg (CGA)	A
	Leu (CUG)	Pro (CCG)	Gln (CAG)	Arg (CGG)	G
A	Ile (AUU)	Thr (ACU)	Asn (AAU)	Ser (AGU)	U
	Ile (AUC)	Thr (ACC)	Asn (AAC)	Ser (AGC)	C
	Ile (AUA)	Thr (ACA)	Lys (AAA)	Arg (AGA)	A
	Met (AUG)	Thr (ACG)	Lys (AAG)	Arg (AGG)	G
G	Val (GUU)	Ala (GCU)	Asp (GAU)	Gly (GGU)	U
	Val (GUC)	Ala (GCC)	Asp (GAC)	Gly (GGC)	C
	Val (GUA)	Ala (GCA)	Glu (GAA)	Gly (GGA)	A
	Val (GUG)	Ala (GCG)	Glu (GAG)	Gly (GGG)	G

Genes carry the code for the amino acids in polypeptide chains. The genetic code is the same in all organisms.

The genetic code

The 20 amino acids [alanine (Ala), arginine (Arg), asparagine (Asn), aspartic acid (Asp), cysteine (Cys), glutamine (Gln), glutamic acid (Glu), glycine (Gly), histidine (His), isoleucine (Ile), leucine (Leu), lysine (Lys), methionine (Met), phenylalanine (Phe), proline (Pro), serine (Ser), threonine (Thr), tryptophan (Trp), tyrosine (Tyr) and valine (Val)] are encoded by base triplets. UAA, UAG and UGA cause termination of transcription.

Gene transcription: transmitting the code

RNA transcription can be divided into stages of:
• initiation;
• elongation;
• termination.

As with DNA replication, the process of gene transcription is more fully understood in prokaryotic than in eukaryotic organisms. This in part reflects the simpler nature of prokaryotic genomes, which consist of closely packed genes, in which the coding DNA sequences are rarely interrupted.

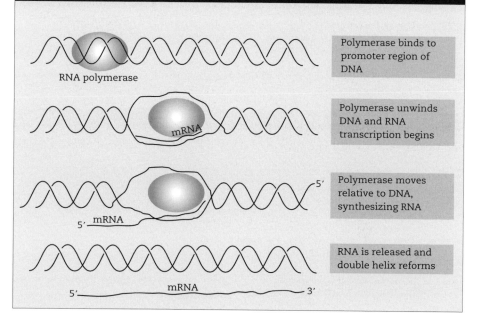

TRANSCRIPTION IN PROKARYOTES

RNA polymerase

Polymerase binds to promoter region of DNA

mRNA

Polymerase unwinds DNA and RNA transcription begins

5′ mRNA

5′

Polymerase moves relative to DNA, synthesizing RNA

RNA is released and double helix reforms

5′ mRNA 3′

Fig. 1.10 Transcription in prokaryotes.

Prokaryotic gene transcription

Gene transcription in prokaryotic cells (Fig. 1.10) is relatively simple.

• *Initiation*. RNA Pol binds to a specific sequence, known as a promoter, which lies just upstream of the coding sequence of the gene.

• *Elongation*. RNA Pol then proceeds through the gene, synthesizing a RNA chain which is a copy of the antisense strand of DNA. The reaction is similar to the polymerization of DNA (see p. 12), in that nucleotide triphosphates are hydrolysed releasing pyrophosphate which is split into inorganic phosphate.

• *Termination*. When the polymerase encounters a specific sequence, known as a terminator, transcription stops and the completed RNA molecule is released.

Gene structure and transcription in eukaryotic cells

Differences in both gene structure and the RNA Pol molecules make transcription in eukaryotes more complex.

In eukaryotic cells:

• there are three different types of RNA Pol (see p. 46);

• transcription is regulated by numerous different proteins, most of which bind to specific sites around the coding region of the gene;

• RNA is modified in several ways before being ready for translation into protein.

Only a small fraction of the human genome encodes polypeptides; over 95% is non-coding with no known function. Non-coding DNA occurs both within and between genes. Some of this apparently functionless DNA contains repetitive sequences of bases, which may be of functional significance. For example, centromeres which ensure complete disjunction at the middle of chromosomes, and telomeres which allow complete replication at the ends of chromosomes, both contain arrays of tandemly repeated DNA.

The structure of eukaryotic genes is more complex than a series of codons. The transcriptional unit of a gene is the region transcribed into a primary RNA transcript, which is a precursor of mRNA. It is made up of exons

CENTROMERES, TELOMERES AND ARRAYS

The *centromere* is the site at which chromosomes constrict during metaphase. It separates the long and short arms of the chromosome.

The *telomere* forms the end of the chromosome.

In *tandemly repeated arrays* identical DNA sequences appear one after the other along a stretch of DNA.

TRANSCRIPTION UNIT

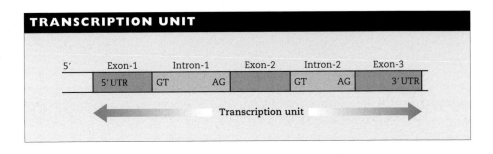

Fig. 1.11 Diagrammatic representation of a eukaryotic transcription unit. UTR, untranslated region.

(containing expressed or coding DNA), which are interrupted by sequences of unknown function known as *intervening sequences* (IVS) or *introns* (Fig. 1.11).

Introns begin with GT and end with AG.

The coding regions in the first and last exons are flanked by untranslated regions (UTRs), which are actually part of the exons and are transcribed into mRNA but not translated into protein.

Sequences on the 5′ side of a region of DNA (to the left in a 5′–3′ sequence) are often called 'upstream', whereas those on the 3′ side are 'downstream'.

The rate at which genes are transcribed is regulated by DNA sequences that usually lie outside the transcription unit, but on the same DNA strand. They tend to occur close to the gene, but may be located thousands of base pairs away.

DNA sequences that influence the transcription of genes are known as *cis-acting control elements*. They do not encode proteins, but often influence gene transcription by acting as binding sites for protein produced by other genes, known as *trans-acting transcription factors* or *DNA-binding proteins*. The mechanism by which such DNA-binding proteins influence gene transcription is not fully understood. It is possible that unfolding or folding of DNA to expose or hide certain sequences, or changes in the position of DNA with respect to the nuclear membrane, may be important.

cis-acting control regions are usually organized in clusters, which are located in the *promoter* and *enhancer* regions of the gene.

Certain DNA sequences are found in the *promoter region* of most genes (Fig. 1.12). These include the TATA and CAAT boxes.
• *TATA box*. Consists of an AT-rich sequence (often TATAA) which occurs about 30 bp upstream from the transcriptional start site (often denoted −30: the position of the nucleotide at the start site is designated +1). TATA boxes are often absent from the promoters of 'housekeeping genes'. Housekeeping genes,

TRANSCRIPTION AND CONTROL REGIONS

The promoter region is located immediately upstream of the gene-coding region and contains sequences that govern the rate of transcription, and define the site at which it starts.

Enhancer/silencer regions may be located within, near or some distance away from the gene whose expression they stimulate, or sometimes suppress.

Structures which facilitate the binding of proteins to DNA have been identified. For example, *zinc fingers* consist of a fold of about 30 amino acids around a zinc atom, which seems to insert into grooves in the DNA helix. *Leucine zippers* contain four or five leucine residues, each one spaced exactly seven residues apart. Pairs of DNA-binding proteins can attach to the 'zipper', and the whole structure then appears to grip the DNA helix, bringing the DNA-binding proteins into contact with their binding domains.

CONTROL REGION

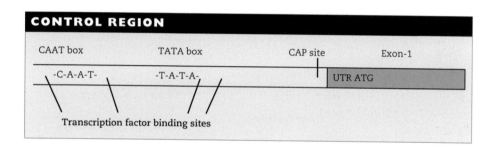

Fig. 1.12 The promotor region of a gene.

such as genes encoding the structural protein actin, are continuously expressed at low levels, and often have GC-rich sequences such as GGGCGG in their promoter regions.

• *CAAT box*. Contains this short sequence about 80 bp upstream (−80) of the start site.

These sequences, together with binding sites for other transcription factors which vary according to the gene involved, are responsible for the rate of transcription.

Transcription starts at the *CAP site*, so called because following transcription, the 5′ end of the mRNA is capped at this site by the attachment of a specialized nucleotide (7-methyl guanosine). The cap site is followed by a *leader sequence* leading up to the *initiation codon* (ATG), that specifies the start of translation.

Transcription then proceeds, such that a full copy of the gene (*introns* and *exons*) is made using a process similar to DNA replication (Fig. 1.13). A *stop codon* (TAA, TAG or TGA) indicates the end of the translated region (Fig. 1.14). This is followed by a UTR, which includes the *poly(A) signal* (AATAAA), that signals cleavage of the newly formed RNA at a position slightly downstream, and the addition of a string of adenylate residues (a poly(A) tail). The poly(A) tail is thus not encoded by the gene; rather adenosine monophosphate residues are sequentially added enzymatically following transcription.

Thus, each end of the mRNA contains a UTR which is not translated into protein. The function of these regions is not fully understood, although the 5′ region (upstream) appears to influence translation, whereas the 3′ region (downstream) may contain sequences that are important in the stability of mRNA.

The 5′ cap binds to the small subunit of the ribosome as the first step in translation.

EUKARYOTIC TRANSCRIPTION

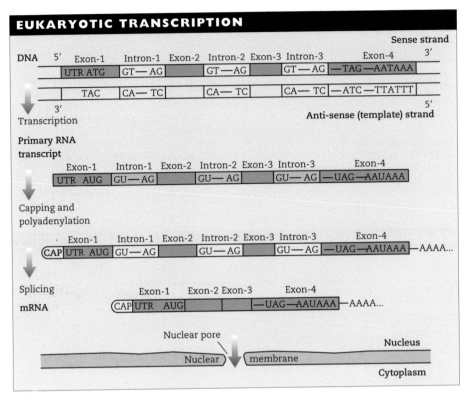

Fig. 1.13 Transcription in a eukaryotic cell.

TERMINATION OF TRANSCRIPTION

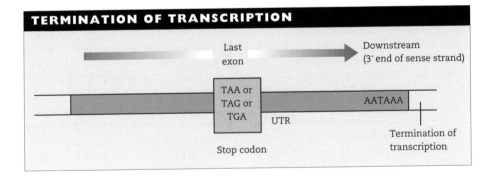

Fig. 1.14 Termination of eukaryotic transcription.

which RNA Pol II is principally involved in transcription of mRNA.

In eukaryotic cells, transcription is mostly controlled at the level of initiation. The binding of transcription factors to the promoter region of a gene attracts RNA Pol. Three types of RNA Pol (I, II and III) occur in eukaryotes, of

The primary RNA transcripts produced by RNA Pol II are referred to as heterogeneous nuclear RNA (hnRNA), because unlike tRNA and rRNA, they show considerable variability (heterogeneity) in size.

ALTERNATIVE SPLICING

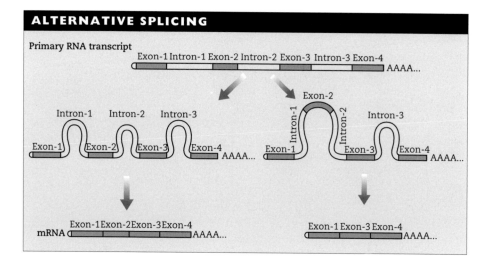

Fig. 1.15 Alternative splicing produces different mRNAs from the same primary transcript.

The presence of proteins which act as transcription factors is required before a RNA Pol II molecule can recognize and bind to the promoter of a gene and start transcription. These are referred to using the prefix TFII (e.g. TFIIA, TFIIB, TFIID, TFIIE, TFIIF, TFIIH in order of their discovery) because they each act as *transcription factors* for RNA Pol II. TFIID binds to the TATA box and is also known as the TATA factor.

Binding of RNA Pol II to the promoter region of a gene results in a localized separation of double-stranded DNA. During formation of an mRNA molecule about 20 bp of DNA are unwound at any one time, of which around 10 form a DNA/RNA hybrid. The RNA Pol proceeds through the gene and synthesizes an mRNA chain from the 5′ to 3′ end by adding ribonucleoside monophosphate bases complementary to the DNA. Only one strand (the antisense strand) is used as a template. The primary RNA transcript is thus an exact copy of the sense DNA strand, except that U replaces T.

Most rRNA is transcribed by RNA Pol I in the nucleolus, whereas the small (5S) rRNA and tRNA are transcribed by RNA Pol III in the extranucleolar region.

Post-transcriptional processing

Whilst still in the nucleus the newly synthesized RNA is modified by the following events.
• *Capping*—the addition of a nucleotide cap.
• *Polyadenylation*—detachment of the RNA and addition of a string of adenosine residues.
• *Splicing*—sequences corresponding to *introns* are *excised* and discarded, and the remaining *exons* are *spliced together*.

During splicing all of the introns are usually removed, leaving all of the exons in the mRNA. However, exons may also be removed during the splicing process, resulting in variations in the final mRNA product, and hence in the polypeptide it encodes. The process by which different mRNA transcripts are formed by removal of different segments of the primary RNA transcript is known as alternative splicing (Fig. 1.15).

After capping, polyadenylation and splicing, the RNA is then ready for transport to the cytoplasm.

Translation: reading the code

Protein synthesis occurs on ribosomes. In eukaryotes, ribosomes consist of 40S (small) and 60S (large) subunits, which together

tRNA

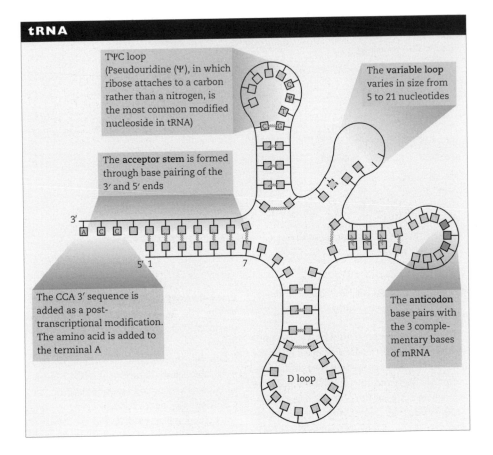

TΨC loop (Pseudouridine (Ψ), in which ribose attaches to a carbon rather than a nitrogen, is the most common modified nucleoside in tRNA)

The acceptor stem is formed through base pairing of the 3′ and 5′ ends

The variable loop varies in size from 5 to 21 nucleotides

The CCA 3′ sequence is added as a post-transcriptional modification. The amino acid is added to the terminal A

The anticodon base pairs with the 3 comple-mentary bases of mRNA

D loop

Fig. 1.16 The structure of tRNA.

form 80S particles (S = Svedberg units, see p. 11). 60S subunits contain proteins complexed to three rRNAs (28S, 5.8S and 5S), whereas in the 40S subunit proteins are complexed to 18S RNA.

The structure of the 30S (small) and 50S (large) subunits of bacterial ribosomes have been resolved at an atomic level. The 30S subunit contains the mRNA decoding site. There are three binding sites for transfer RNA (Fig. 1.16). These are the A (acceptor), P (peptidyl) and E (exit) sites. These three sites are involved in the selection of tRNA, the addition

of the amino acid it carries to the growing amino acid chain, and the completion of polypeptide synthesis (Fig. 1.17).

The process of protein synthesis is started by the formation of a complex involving the small ribosomal subunit carrying a methionine tRNA, which base pairs with the initiation codon AUG on mRNA (Fig. 1.16).

Once the initiation complex has formed, synthesis of the polypeptide chain is driven by elongation factors (eIFs), which join the large subunit to the complex and move the ribosome relative to the mRNA.

Each tRNA carries an amino acid and a triplet of bases (anticodon), which recognize a codon on mRNA specific for the amino acid. For example, the tRNA that carries

TRANSLATION: MAKING PROTEINS

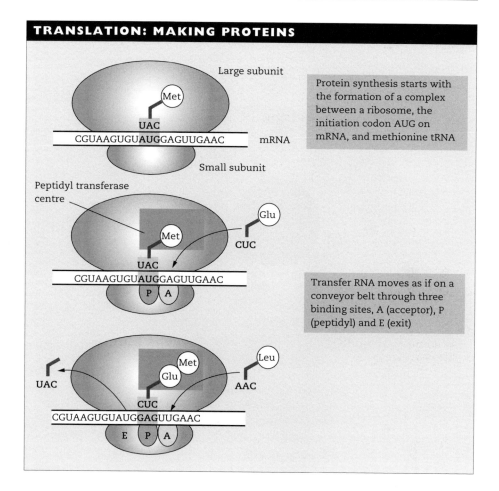

Large subunit

Small subunit

mRNA

Protein synthesis starts with the formation of a complex between a ribosome, the initiation codon AUG on mRNA, and methionine tRNA

Peptidyl transferase centre

Transfer RNA moves as if on a conveyor belt through three binding sites, A (acceptor), P (peptidyl) and E (exit)

Fig. 1.17 Translating the genetic code of mRNA into the polypeptide chain of a protein.

methionine has the anticodon UAC which recognizes the methionine codon AUG on mRNA. The peptidyl transferase reaction that joins amino acids together is catalysed by RNA molecules which are exposed on the surface of the ribosome by the folded structure it adopts. Thus the ribosome is a ribozyme.

When the ribosome reaches a termination codon (UAA, UAG or UGA) the com-

RIBOZYMES

Some RNA molecules are able to function as enzymes. These catalytic RNA molecules are known as ribozymes. They were initially identified by their ability to cleave RNA. The ribosome contains RNA molecules that catalyse the formation of peptide bonds that join amino acids during protein synthesis.

pleted polypeptide is released from the last tRNA, and the ribosomal units fall off the mRNA.

DIAGRAM OF A CELL

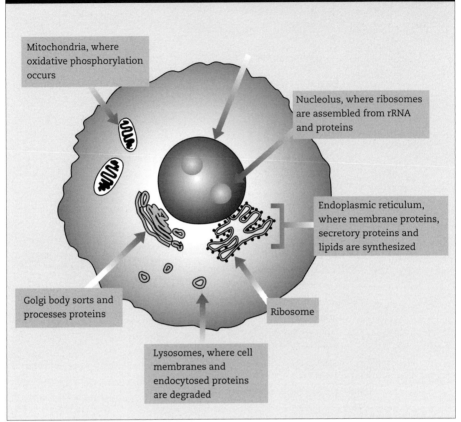

Mitochondria, where oxidative phosphorylation occurs

Nucleolus, where ribosomes are assembled from rRNA and proteins

Endoplasmic reticulum, where membrane proteins, secretory proteins and lipids are synthesized

Golgi body sorts and processes proteins

Ribosome

Lysosomes, where cell membranes and endocytosed proteins are degraded

Fig. 1.18 Representation of a eukaryotic cell showing some of the important organelles.

Post-translational processing

Polypeptides may start to form the complex structure of proteins as they are synthesized.

Secretory proteins pass through the rough endoplasmic reticulum and move to the Golgi body for processing (Fig. 1.18). Following synthesis many polypeptides are modified further, e.g. by hydroxylation or phosphorylation of amino acids, or addition of sugars (glycosylation).

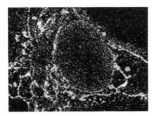

Biomolecular Tools

Molecular medicine is based on the ability to manipulate biological molecules. Technologies for manipulating the nucleic acids DNA and RNA are extensive and protein technology is developing rapidly. This chapter provides an overview of the technologies involved, with an emphasis on understanding some of the fundamental principles that underlie the rapidly evolving techniques. The basic procedures and important enzymes are introduced, along with how these tools are used to answer specific questions. Such background will improve your understanding of current research findings. A better grasp of the fundamental technology will also help in appreciating the possibilities and identifying the limits of gene technology.

Performing these increasingly complex techniques is challenging and they can be adopted by many laboratories only because of the availability of excellent reagents and kits. There is also a trend to 'outsource' to commercial enterprises or institutional core facilities some procedures, especially those requiring particular skills or expensive instruments. Even if 'cloning by phoning' is your approach, understanding the fundamentals will help you decide whom to call.

Nucleic acid preparation and analysis

The relative structural simplicity and homogeneity of nucleic acids led many early researchers to doubt that DNA *could* be the 'stuff' of which genes are made. Nucleic acids were wrongly thought to be merely structural elements of chromosomes, perhaps organizing the proteins that were deemed complicated enough to constitute genes. The fact that genes are composed of only four biochemically similar nucleotides, which convey information in their sequence and not their tertiary structure, makes the chemistry of isolation and characterization correspondingly uniform, i.e. independent of their sequence.

Nucleic acids are uniformly and strongly negatively charged because of their phosphate backbones (see Chapter 1). Therefore, they prefer an aqueous environment where these charges are hydrated. Other cellular constituents, such as proteins, lipids and carbohydrates, contain charged and uncharged regions as well as hydrophobic and hydrophilic regions, which make these molecules prefer either a hydrophobic (organic) environment or the interface between organic and aqueous phases. This is the basis of extraction by the organic solvent phenol and other separations. Nucleic acids are also relatively dense and can therefore be separated on caesium chloride (CsCl) gradients.

The ways in which DNA and RNA *differ*, and how these differences are exploited in their purification, will be described next, before embarking on a discussion of their manipulation.

DNA preparation

DNA is easy to prepare and store, principally because DNA-specific degrading enzymes (DNases) are easily destroyed by moderate heating (65°C) or inhibited by compounds that sequester (chelate) divalent ions, such as ethylene diamine tetra-acetic acid (EDTA). For some purposes, such as preparing a template for the polymerase chain reaction (PCR), it is sufficient simply to lyse the cells (i.e. destroy the cells through rupture of the plasma membrane) and denature the proteins and DNA at high temperature (95°C).

When native (double-stranded) DNA or purer preparations are required, protein can be extracted by phenol or separated by centrifugation through a density gradient formed by CsCl solutions.

Chromosomal DNA: long and stringy

Chromosomal (genomic) DNA is difficult to prepare without shearing (tearing apart) at

least some of the DNA. This is hardly surprising when one considers that the DNA contained in one mammalian cell is nearly 2 m long (stretched end to end and deprived of packaging proteins), so the DNA from even a few cells can produce quite a knot. Even the much shorter chromosomal DNA from bacteria (~1 mm) can become a mess quickly and irreversibly.

When large pieces of DNA (> 50 000 bp) are needed intact, as when mapping genes by pulsed field gel electrophoresis (PFGE, see p. 33), cells can be first embedded in a gel. They are then lysed, protein is removed, and the DNA digested right in the gel (*in situ*). This avoids manipulation that could shear long pieces of DNA. Fortunately, it is rare that very large pieces of DNA are analysed intact. The more common, practical problem is that chromosomal DNA is extremely difficult to transfer from one tube to another because it is so stringy (viscous).

Plasmid DNA: small and circular

Plasmids are small, circular DNAs that are extrachromosomal and independently replicating in bacteria because they have their own origin of replication (*ori*). Bacteria have always exchanged useful genes using plasmids; molecular biologists have caught on only in the last couple of decades. Plasmids are quite easy to isolate from bacteria, manipulate *in vitro* and reintroduce into bacteria. Therefore, they are often used as *cloning vectors*, meaning that desired DNA is inserted into the plasmid and then 'grown up' along with the rest of the plasmid DNA.

Using recombinant DNA techniques, plasmids have been improved for use as cloning vectors in the following ways (Fig. 2.1).
• Addition of restriction enzyme sites that allow the plasmid to be cut at particular sites (e.g. the polylinker).
• Addition of genes that allow simpler screening and selection procedures to find successful recombinants (e.g. *lacZ'*).
• Removal of DNA to make the plasmid smaller and deletion of restriction enzyme

DENATURATION

Biological molecules have a natural configuration that is necessary for their activity. When this native configuration is disturbed or destroyed, the molecule is said to be *denatured*. For proteins, the configuration is determined during initial folding by the interaction of smaller structural elements such as sheets, coils and helices. For DNA, the principal structural element is its double-stranded nature. Thus, DNA is denatured when it is made single stranded and renatured when the double strand is reformed. RNA is a single strand that folds to form double-stranded regions. RNA is denatured when these regions are made single stranded.

PLASMID ANATOMY

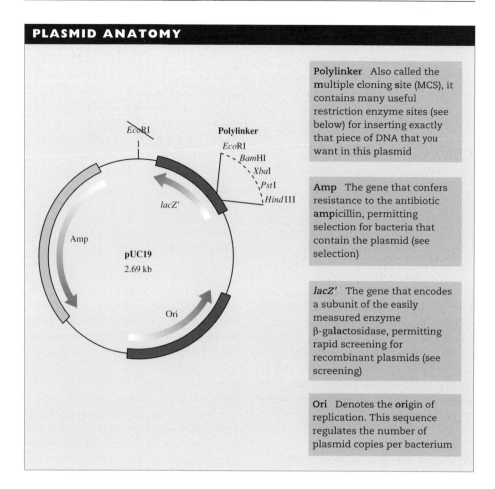

Polylinker Also called the multiple cloning site (MCS), it contains many useful restriction enzyme sites (see below) for inserting exactly that piece of DNA that you want in this plasmid

Amp The gene that confers resistance to the antibiotic **ampicillin**, permitting selection for bacteria that contain the plasmid (see selection)

lacZ' The gene that encodes a subunit of the easily measured enzyme β-galactosidase, permitting rapid screening for recombinant plasmids (see screening)

Ori Denotes the origin of replication. This sequence regulates the number of plasmid copies per bacterium

Fig. 2.1 Plasmids are the workhorses of molecular biology. For example, the plasmid pUC19 is a second-generation, relatively simple, cloning vector of 2686 bp (2.7 kb) that was constructed from parts of earlier plasmids using recombinant DNA technology.

sites (e.g. the *Eco*RI site formerly at position 1), which makes the plasmid easier to manipulate.
• Substitution of a mutant origin of replication (*ori*) that allows *relaxed copy number* control, meaning that the plasmid continues to replicate after the bacterium has stopped. Although not desirable for the bacterium or the symbiotic plasmid, this is great for producing a much higher yield of DNA for the molecular biologist.

Plasmid DNA can be transferred into mammalian cells through a process called *transfection*. The transfected plasmid is usually lost after a few rounds of cell division but it can occasionally become incorporated into genomic DNA, producing a stable transfectant. There are also plasmids that include pieces of animal viruses such as SV40 (simian virus 40) or retroviruses that enable their autonomous replication in mammalian cells. Yeast and mammals also have natural circular, independently replicating, extrachromosomal DNAs (e.g. mitochondrial DNA), but they are larger, do not possess multiple cloning sites, screening or selection functions, and do not replicate in bacteria, so they lack many of the attributes of a good cloning vector.

PLASMIDS ARE CIRCULAR

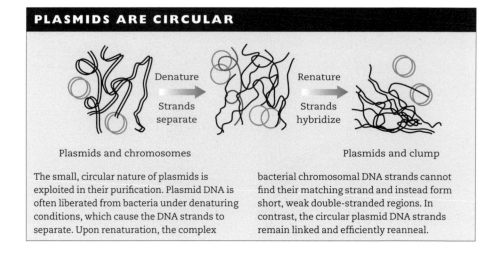

Denature
Strands separate

Renature
Strands hybridize

Plasmids and chromosomes

The small, circular nature of plasmids is exploited in their purification. Plasmid DNA is often liberated from bacteria under denaturing conditions, which cause the DNA strands to separate. Upon renaturation, the complex

Plasmids and clump

bacterial chromosomal DNA strands cannot find their matching strand and instead form short, weak double-stranded regions. In contrast, the circular plasmid DNA strands remain linked and efficiently reanneal.

Plasmids are often named with a p (for plasmid) followed by identifying letters (often the initials of the designer) and the edition number. Numbering of the base pairs starts at the top marked 'I' and proceeds clockwise. During the construction of pUC19 (Fig. 2.1), an *EcoRI* restriction enzyme site that was originally at this position was deleted, as indicated by the line through the name, to maintain a unique *EcoRI* site in the polylinker.

cDNA (complementary DNA)

cDNA stands for *complementary DNA*, which means DNA that is synthesized as the opposite or complementary strand of messenger RNA (mRNA). To make cDNA, RNA is first prepared and then reverse transcribed (see also *Reverse transcriptase*, p. 48).

RNA preparation

RNA takes several different forms (Table 2.1). RNA preparation is difficult because ribonucleases (RNases, enzymes that degrade RNA) are extremely stable and can even refold and regain activity after complete denaturation. Therefore, methods of isolating RNA attempt to:

1 inhibit cellular RNases;
2 separate RNA from DNA and proteins (including RNases); and
3 keep RNase out.

Many protocols employ lysis buffers containing guanidinium, which is a strong protein denaturant and a strong inhibitor of RNases. The problem with guanidinium is that it also inhibits nearly everything else. Therefore, the residual guanidinium is often reduced by ethanol precipitating the RNA (see p. 30) before treatment with enzymes.

Aside from the cells themselves, fingers are an important source of RNases. Wearing gloves may help, but they can quickly become contaminated with RNase after handling pipettes, bottles, etc. Great care must be taken in preparing materials. Tubes and pipette tips are often autoclaved or baked to destroy RNase. Some solutions can be treated with diethylpyrocarbonate (DEPC), which irreversibly denatures RNases, and then autoclaved to destroy the DEPC. However, residual DEPC can interfere with analysis and many solutions cannot be treated with DEPC because it reacts with the solute. Therefore, use of caution and the purest possible solutions is often the best approach. RNases can be also specifically inhibited with *RNasin* (*RNase inhibitor*), an easily denatured (labile) protein that is relatively expensive but also effective and safe.

Although ribosomal RNA (rRNA) is rarely specifically prepared, its presence in most RNA preparations is useful. It acts as a carrier for the rarer mRNA and it produces strong,

Table 2.1 RNA takes many forms, which perform distinct functions and are prepared differently.

RNA TYPES AND THEIR PREPARATION

RNA name (aliases)	What is it?	How much is there?	How is it prepared?
Total	All the RNA in the cell	~1% of cell mass	Guanidinium lysis, then phenol extraction or CsCl ultracentrifugation
Cytoplasmic	Non-nuclear	Most of the total	Lysis with low detergent concentrations, which keeps nucleus intact; purify RNA from cytoplasm
Messenger (mRNA) (poly A⁺)	RNA possessing a 'tail' of A nucleotides	Very little (3% total) Naturally, the most desirable	Prepare total or cytoplasmic RNA, purify poly(A) ('annealing and elute by denaturing the RNA Extremely heterogeneous in size
Ribosomal (rRNA)	Structural components of ribosomes	Most of the total RNA	Only rarely Four sizes: 28S (4718 5S (120 bp)
Transfer (tRNA)	Adapters between mRNA and amino acids	Plenty	Only rarely About 100 different forms, 75

easily detectable bands when total or cytoplasmic RNA preparations are analysed by gel electrophoresis, which separates molecules by size (see Fig. 2.4). The heterogeneously sized mRNA produces only a faint smear on gels. The sharpness and relative intensities of two main rRNA bands are good indicators of the mRNA quality and quantity. Mammalian rRNA produces two prominent bands of lengths 4718 and 1874 bp, called 28S and 18S, respectively. (S is for Svedberg, the unit of measurement for speed of sedimentation upon ultracentrifugation.) If these bands are sharp and the 28S band is about twice as bright as the 18S band, then the RNA preparation has probably not suffered significant digestion by RNases. Although the smaller 5.8S (160-bp) and 5S (120-bp) rRNAs are present in equal numbers (they are all subunits of the ribosome), their small size makes them relatively difficult to detect on gels.

Nucleic acid measurement and manipulation

Optical density (OD) measurement: how much, how pure?

Nucleotides in solution absorb light in the ultraviolet (UV) region of the spectrum, with a maximum absorption around a wavelength of 260 nm (Table 2.2). Proteins also absorb UV light, but more at the 280 nm wavelength and less at 260 nm (Fig. 2.2). Therefore, nucleic acids can be quantified and the purity of a preparation can be estimated by measuring the absorption at both 260 and 280 nm (spectrophotometry) and comparing the results to those obtained from pure solutions. The term OD is commonly used instead of absorbance.

The OD at additional wavelengths may be measured to determine the extent of contamination by chemicals used in the preparation. For example, phenol contamination can be estimated from the OD 270, whereas guanidinium contamination can be estimated at OD 230, although many other compounds also absorb at these wavelengths (Fig. 2.2).

The OD values are used to determine the amount and purity of a DNA or RNA preparation. For example, if protein is present in the solution, the OD 280 increases more than the OD 260 (because proteins absorb light of 280 nm wavelength better than 260 nm), so the ratio OD 260/OD 280 decreases. Pure DNA has a ratio of OD 260/OD 280 of 1.8, while pure RNA has a ratio of 2.0.

Ethanol precipitation

DNA and RNA can be efficiently precipitated (made insoluble) by adding salt and alcohol and

---

QUANTITATION OF NUCLEOTIDES: LIGHT! CAMERA! MEASURE!

	Deoxynucleotides			
	dATP	dTTP	dGTP	dCTP
OD 260*	1.52	0.84	1.20	0.71

* Shorthand for: 'The optical density at a wavelength of 260 nm of a 0.1 mmol/L solution of this nucleotide is . . .'
dATP, deoxyadenosine triphosphate; dCTP, deoxycytidine triphosphate; dGTP, deoxyguanosine triphosphate; dTTP, deoxythymidine triphosphate

Table 2.2 Different nucleotides absorb different amounts of light. For each nucleotide, the optical density (OD) at 260 nm of a 0.1 mM (100 µmol/L) solution is listed. These values are useful for determining the concentrations of nucleotides or shorter oligonucleotides. Note that the absorbances of the two pyrimidines (cytosine and thymine) and the two purines (adenine and guanine) are similar to each other, so differences in nucleotide composition (percentage of guanine/cytosine) has less effect on OD.

MEASUREMENT OF NUCLEIC ACIDS AND CONTAMINANTS

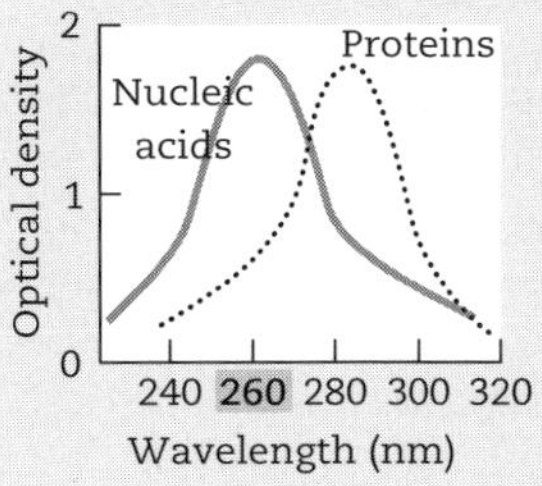

Measure what?	Where?
Nucleic acid (mostly)	260 nm
For pure DNA at 50 µg/ml, OD 260 = 1	
For pure RNA at 40 µg/ml, OD 260 = 1	
Protein (mostly)	280 nm
Contaminants	
Guanidinium, etc.	230 nm
Phenol, etc.	270 nm

Fig. 2.2 Optical density (OD) measurement at different wavelengths helps to determine what is in a solution. Nucleotides absorb ultraviolet light with a maximum at 260 nm. The OD value is dimensionless because it is a ratio of the light absorbed by the experimental sample versus an empty solution.

HYPOCHROMICITY

A couple of quick calculations would suggest that the observed OD values shown above are inconsistent.

A solution of *nucleotides* with an OD 260 of $1 \div 1.07$ (average nucleotide OD 260/0.1 mM, Table 2.2) = 0.093 mM nucleotides.

A solution of *DNA* with an OD 260 of 1 = 50 µg/mL × 1 µmol/330 µg (average molecular weight, Fig. 2.2) = 0.152 mM nucleotides.

This effect is called *hypochromicity*, which probably occurs because the nucleotides in double-stranded DNA are stacked, placing many in their neighbours' shadow where they cannot absorb all the UV light that they would if they were single. Therefore, one should calculate the amount of double-stranded DNA using the observed (hypochromatic) values and the amount of shorter oligonucleotides using the ODs of the individual nucleotides.

centrifuging. The addition of salt increases the ionic strength of the aqueous solution, which reduces the repulsion of the like-charged (negatively charged) phosphate groups on the nucleic acid backbone, thereby allowing the nucleic acid molecules to come closer

together. The addition of alcohol makes the solution more hydrophobic and therefore less able to solvate the charged nucleic acid. These effects combine to reduce the solubility of the nucleic acids and produce the precipitate.

The early protocols called for the mixture to be incubated in the cold, which explains why many 'old-timers' still keep their ethanol in the freezer. Careful analysis later found that room temperature incubation is better for standard DNA precipitation. The precipitate is collected by centrifugation and the pellet is dried and then resuspended in the desired buffer. The choice of salt depends on the intended use of the nucleic acid. For example, ammonium acetate precipitation efficiently removes unincorporated nucleotides after labelling nucleic acids adding traceable nucleotides. However, the residual salt can inhibit some enzymes (e.g. polymerases, which add nucleotides, or kinases, which add phosphate) that may be needed in subsequent reactions.

Fluorescent 'staining' of DNA and RNA

Ethidium bromide (2,7-diamino-10-ethyl-9-phenylphenanthridinium bromide, EtBr) is a small molecule that inserts (intercalates) between the nucleotides of DNA or RNA and strongly fluoresces under UV illumination. Fluorescence is a phenomenon where a compound is excited by absorbing light at one wavelength and relaxes by emitting light at a different wavelength. In this case, the exciting UV light is literally invisible and a longer-wavelength, visible light is emitted. This forms the

DNA/RNA PRECIPITATION: A RECIPE

DNA or RNA
+ salt (to taste*)
+ alcohol (in moderation†)

─────────────────────

= precipitated nucleic acid (spin hard‡ to collect)
Nucleic acids can be efficiently precipitated from salt solutions by adding alcohol.

* Sodium chloride or sodium acetate (0.2 M), ammonium acetate (2.5 M) or lithium chloride (0.8 M) are often used.
† Add 2 volumes ethanol for DNA, 2.5 volumes ethanol for RNA or 1 volume 2-propanol (isopropanol).
‡ Centrifuge, spin 10 minutes at ~12 000 × g.

basis of a quick, easy and sensitive detection system or 'stain' of nucleic acids. When EtBr binds to DNA or RNA, it is effectively concentrated and its fluorescence increases, so the nucleic acid shows up as a bright band on a dim background of unbound EtBr.

Newer, improved stains are gradually replacing EtBr. For example, a stain called SYBR Green I fluoresces more brightly than EtBr upon binding DNA, is practically non-fluorescent in the absence of DNA, and is specific for double-stranded DNA. Methylene blue also stains DNA, is visible under normal lighting conditions, and does not inhibit enzymes that act on DNA. These dyes are also said to be less mutagenic than EtBr.

Fig. 2.3 Molecules of different sizes can be separated on columns or gels. Note that the order of separation is reversed: larger molecules pass more quickly through the column but more slowly through the gel.

Gels and columns: separation by size

Gels and sizing columns separate molecules in opposite order: small molecules come out of a gel *first* and out of a column *last*. This is because a gel is a mesh that large molecules have a relatively hard time getting through, whereas columns contain beads with small pores that exclude large molecules, but allow in small molecules (Fig. 2.3). Since the small molecules can enter the beads, the volume of the column is bigger for them, whereas the excluded large molecules 'see' only the volume between the beads. This is called the *void volume* because it is made up from the voids left between the beads that pack the column. Therefore, larger molecules come out (elute) in a smaller volume (earlier).

The fluid in both columns and gels usually contains a buffer chosen to resist changes in pH. Molecules move through a column in the bulk flow of fluid, driven by gravity or by a pump. In contrast, molecules are driven

SEPARATION OF MOLECULES—BIG ONES FIRST, OR LAST

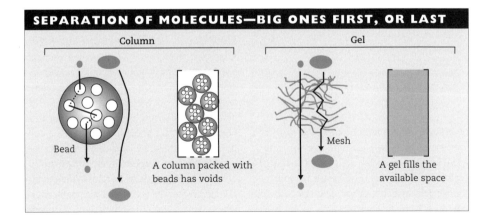

Column   Gel

Bead

A column packed with beads has voids

Mesh

A gel fills the available space

GEL ANALYSIS OF DNA: HOW MUCH? HOW BIG?

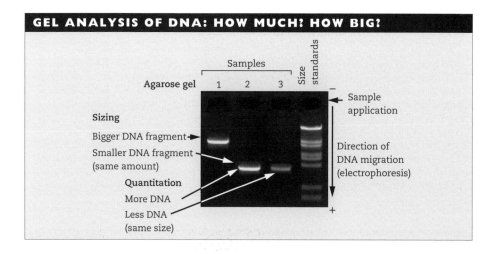

Fig. 2.4 Analysis of DNA by agarose gel electrophoresis allows the estimation of size and quantity. The DNA is detected with a fluorescent ethidium bromide 'stain'.

through a gel by a voltage gradient. DNA and RNA are uniformly negatively charged and naturally adopt a stretched, rod-like configuration. This means that sieving of nucleic acids is a function of their length, unlike proteins that normally fold up compactly and have to be denatured with anionic detergent to be resolved according to polypeptide chain length.

DNA is negatively charged at neutral pH so it migrates toward the positively charged electrode. The discrete size fragments are usually called 'bands'. Note that the *amount* of DNA in a band, not the size of the DNA in a band, determines the amount of EtBr bound and the resulting fluorescence (Fig. 2.4). Confusion on this point is perhaps a consequence of the typical experiment in which a particular DNA is digested and the resulting fragments are analysed by gel electrophoresis. Equal numbers of smaller and larger fragments are generated. However, any particular larger fragment fluoresces brighter than a smaller fragment because it has more base pairs per molecule and comprises more mass. An example of such a digestion is in the right lane of Fig. 2.4, labelled 'Size standards'.

Nucleic acids are often detected in the gel stained with EtBr and illuminated by UV light (Fig. 2.4). This stain can detect as little as 1 ng of DNA in a single band. EtBr is mutagenic and toxic, so solutions and gels must be handled with gloves and disposed of properly. Also, UV light can burn the retina and the skin. Gloves and UV-blocking safety glasses are worn when DNA fragments resolved on gels are prepared. EtBr combined with UV light also damages DNA and RNA, so exposure of the sample should be minimized.

Really big pieces of DNA, such as even a relatively small piece of a chromosome, cannot be separated by conventional gel electrophoresis. This is probably because the DNA begins to snake through the gel and only small differences are seen in the movements of short versus long snakes. Pulsed field gel electrophoresis (PFGE) was developed to separate large pieces of DNA. The voltage gradient (field) is periodically reorientated so that large pieces of DNA cannot remain orientated 'end-on' and separation by size is possible.

Purification on caesium chloride gradients: density is destiny

RNA is denser than DNA, which in turn is denser than the other cellular material that you do not want (protein, lipids, polysaccharides, etc.). So, whilst RNA sinks below a dense

METHODS OF SEPARATION OVER COLUMNS

In addition to sizing columns, which are also called molecular sieves, there are columns that separate molecules by other characteristics. These techniques evolved to separate colour dyes hence are often referred to as *chromatography*.

For example:
- Ion-exchange chromatography separates molecules by their *charge*. This is the basis of popular DNA and RNA preparation kits using disposable, anion exchange columns.

- Affinity chromatography separates molecules by their specific, shape-dependent *binding* to the column material.
- Reversed-phase chromatography separates molecules by their *hydrophobicity (aversion to water)*.

A form of gel electrophoresis called isoelectric focusing (IEF) also separates molecules by their net charge. Although these are powerful analytical techniques, they are used much less often than sizing columns or gels.

PURIFICATION OF NUCLEIC ACIDS BY DENSITY

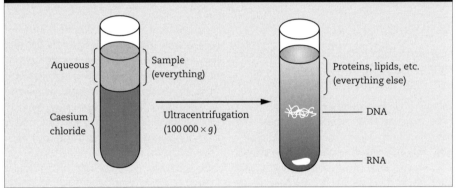

Fig. 2.5 Nucleic acids can be purified through caesium chloride (CsCl) gradients. The ethidium bromide (EtBr)-stained nucleic acids fluoresce under UV illumination and appear as bright bands.

solution of caesium chloride (CsCl), DNA stays in the CsCl and the other material floats above the CsCl solution (Fig. 2.5). This separation occurs during ultracentrifugation (100 000 × g) in the presence of EtBr.

A special use of CsCl/ultracentrifugation is to purify plasmids. Most chromosomal and plasmid DNA is naturally negatively supercoiled, meaning that it possesses an extra twist anticlockwise, once every ~200 bp (Fig. 2.6). The maintenance of the supercoiled state in plasmids is dependent upon the integrity of

both DNA strands. A break in one strand (a 'nick') allows the unwinding of the supercoil and the DNA molecule reverts to the lower-energy relaxed form. Note that a single-stranded break results in the covalently closed circular form, whereas juxtaposed double-stranded breaks result in the linear form. Supercoiled DNA molecules are more dense than relaxed circular or linear molecules, so they 'float' lower on the CsCl density gradient.

CsCl density purification in the presence of EtBr complicates the mechanism, but does not change the result. When EtBr intercalates between the nucleotides, it pushes the nucleotides further apart and unwinds the helix, first unwinding the negative supercoils and then inducing positive supercoils (clockwise twists). In a closed (supercoiled) circle there is only a

SUPERCOILED DNA—GENES WRAPPED TIGHT

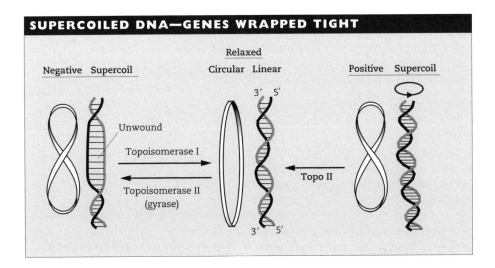

Fig. 2.6 Supercoiled is the natural way. The supercoiled DNA forms a denser structure than relaxed DNA or separate strands. Note that in circular DNA, rotation of strands relative to each other must be some integral number of turns, because half turns juxtapose incompatible ends (3'–3' and 5'–5').

limited amount of intercalation and unwinding that can occur, because the ends of the molecule are fixed. Therefore, the supercoiled plasmids allow only a limited amount of EtBr to

Fig. 2.7 Phenol extracts proteins from aqueous solutions. Near neutral pH, nucleic acids remain in the aqueous phase.

intercalate, remain denser and float relatively lower on the CsCl gradient than the chromosomal DNA.

Phenol extraction: protein removal

Phenol is an organic solvent that is often used to separate nucleic acids and proteins. Phenol is added to the solution of proteins and nucleic acids and the tube is shaken vigorously (often 'vortexed') to mix, then the tube is centrifuged to accelerate the separation of the organic and aqueous phases (Fig. 2.7). If large molecular weight DNA is being prepared, mixing is performed by gently inverting the tube in order to minimize DNA shearing. Proteins are denatured and segregate into the phenol or remain

PHENOL EXTRACTION OF PROTEINS

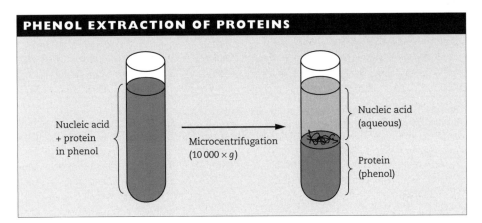

pH-DEPENDENT PARTITIONING OF RNA AND DNA		
Phenol pH	Aqueous phase	Organic phase
Neutral (pH 7–8)	RNA + DNA	Protein, etc.
Acidic (pH 4.8)	RNA	DNA, protein, etc.

Table 2.3 Acidic phenol is used to prepare RNA depleted of DNA.

at the aqueous interface. At near-neutral pH, nucleic acids stay in the aqueous phase because of their highly negatively charged phosphate backbone.

Phenol is toxic, and a notable alternative for the removal of proteins is to make proteins insoluble with high salt concentrations and then to remove the protein precipitate by centrifugation. Because salt, unlike phenol, is not a denaturant, high salt precipitation is not as effective as phenol in removing proteins. However, nucleic acids can be immediately and selectively precipitated out of the protein-depleted high salt solution by the addition of ethanol.

A popular method for extracting RNA uses acidic phenol, which keeps the RNA in the aqueous phase but sends the DNA into the phenol phase, probably because the phosphate groups on the DNA are more easily neutralized (i.e. less acidic) (Table 2.3).

Recombination: designer genes

Restriction enzymes and ligase— cutting and pasting DNA

Restriction endonucleases are enzymes that cut (digest) DNA at specific sequences (sites).

Editing DNA with enzymes

Molecular biology is founded on the ability to cut DNA at specific places, producing fragments that can be recombined in different ways (recombinant DNA). Restriction endonucleases and ligases are the enzymes that perform these functions.

RESTRICTION AND MODIFICATION: BACTERIAL DEFENCE

Restriction enzymes are purified from a variety of bacteria, which use them for defence against viruses called bacteriophages (literally 'bacteria eaters'). Bacteriophage DNA is said to be *restricted* (cut) by a bacterial strain when it cannot infect that strain of bacterium. Bacteria avoid cutting their own genomic DNA by *modifying* it, particularly through methylation, rather than forbidding these DNA sequences. Modification systems vary amongst bacterial strains. Mammalian DNA can usually be cut by restriction enzymes *in vitro* because eukaryotic methylation patterns differ from those of bacteria (prokaryotes). (In eukaryotes, DNA methylation is involved with gene expression and compaction.) Ironically, restriction enzymes allow molecular biologists to generate recombinant DNA plasmids, which they introduce into and grow in bacteria. In the laboratory, bacterial strains mutant in one or more of the *restriction–modification* (R–M) system enzymes are used as hosts to reduce incompatibility problems. All commonly used restriction enzymes are type II, which recognize symmetrical DNA sequences, cut symmetrically, and leave 3'-hydroxyl and 5'-phosphate ends. Type II restriction enzymes are dimers of single polypeptides, which are easier to mass produce than are multisubunit enzymes. The rarely used type I and III restriction enzymes contain multiple subunits. They recognize specific sequences but do not cut exactly or completely.

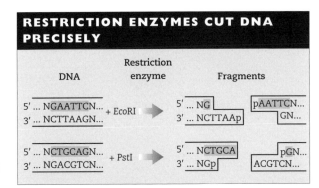

RESTRICTION ENZYMES CUT DNA PRECISELY

Fig. 2.8 Different restriction enzymes cut different sequences. 'N' means any DNA base and only the new terminal phosphate (p) is shown.

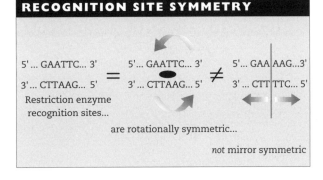

RECOGNITION SITE SYMMETRY

Fig. 2.9 Nearly all commonly used restriction enzymes cut rotationally symmetrical sequences. Recognition sequences are often said to be palindromes, as in the phrase 'Madam, I'm Adam' (in which the comma/apostrophe is rotationally symmetrical).

Restriction enzymes

Restriction endonucleases with over 200 different sequence specificities have been characterized; therefore, many different fragments can be generated. For example, the enzyme *Eco*RI ('echo R one', isolated from *Escherichia coli*) cuts DNA at the sequence GAATTC, whereas *Pst*I (isolated from a different bacterium) cuts at the sequence CTGCAG (Fig. 2.8).

Commonly used restriction enzymes typically recognize symmetrical DNA sequences (Fig. 2.9). This symmetry is a consequence of the fact that these enzymes are homodimers, composed of two identical protein subunits.

Note the importance of the 5'-N-3' orientation as a convention for writing DNA sequences (Fig. 2.10). *Eco*RI, which cuts the sequence 5'-GAATTC, would not cut the same sequence of nucleotides in the opposite orientation (3'-GAATTC). As it happens, the restriction enzyme *Afl*II would cut this sequence (5'-CTTAAG).

The examples given above are all 6-bp recognition sites. The six-base cutters are used most often because they tend to cut DNA into fragments that are small enough to handle yet big enough to be useful. The average fragment length is a function of the size of the recognition sequence and the approximately random distribution of A/T/G/C in DNA (ignoring for now the fact that the mammalian genome is AT-rich and CG-poor). With four bases to choose from, a given sequence of six base pairs occurs once every approximately 4000 bases ($4^6 = 4096$) by chance. In contrast, an 8-bp cutter like *Not*I is more useful for mapping larger pieces of DNA such as mammalian genomes, because it produces only one-sixteenth as many DNA fragments (of an average 64 000 bp).

Over 2000 restriction enzymes have been isolated to date, with around 200 different sequence specificities, which means that there are usually several enzymes that recognize a

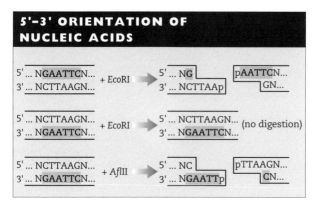

5'-3' ORIENTATION OF NUCLEIC ACIDS

Fig. 2.10 Orientation is important because 5'-GAATTC is not the same as 3'-GAATTC.

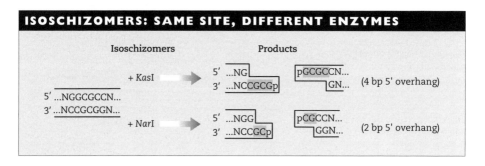

ISOSCHIZOMERS: SAME SITE, DIFFERENT ENZYMES

Fig. 2.11 Isoschizomers are different restriction enzymes that recognize the same sequence but may cut in different ways.

given sequence. When different restriction enzymes recognize the same sequence, they are called *isoschizomers*. They do not always cut at the same place in the sequence (Fig. 2.11).

The frequency of certain restriction enzyme sites is actually much lower than expected. As noted above, mammalian genomes are A- and T-rich, which reduces the frequency of restriction sites containing G or C. Even so, the frequency of the CG dinucleotide is fivefold lower than would be expected based on G and C content alone. Consequently, restriction enzyme sites containing CG are relatively rare in mammalian genomes. Furthermore, these CG sites are often methylated, which is a modification that blocks cutting by many restriction enzymes. Surprisingly, the genome is not homogeneous in this respect: stretches of

several hundred to thousand base pairs, called CG dinucleotide 'islands', are found in which the CG dinucleotide occurs at nearly the expected frequency. Often, these islands are found 5' of genes, an early observation that has since led to the identification and cloning of several genes based solely on their position downstream (3') of CG islands (see Chapter 3).

Ligases

DNA ligase takes two ends and connects the phosphate backbone. Three types of ends can be ligated: blunt, 'sticky', and single-strand nicks.

Sticky ligations are more efficient because the compatible ends stick together (anneal), albeit weakly (Fig. 2.12). On the other hand, blunt-end ligations are particularly useful because of the ability to recombine any DNA fragments,

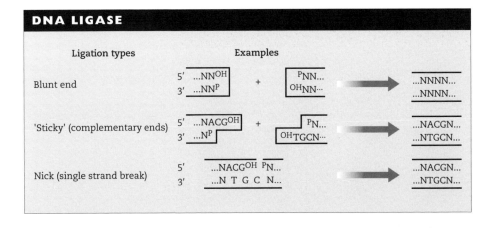

DNA LIGASE

Ligation types	Examples	

Blunt end

$5'$ ...NN^{OH}
$3'$ ...NN^{P} + ^{P}NN...
^{OH}NN...   →   ...NNNN...
...NNNN...

'Sticky' (complementary ends)

$5'$ ...NACG^{OH}
$3'$ ...N^{P} + ^{P}N...
^{OH}TGCN...   →   ...NACGN...
...NTGCN...

Nick (single strand break)

$5'$ ...NACG^{OH} ^{P}N...
$3'$ ...N T G C N...   →   ...NACGN...
...NTGCN...

Fig. 2.12 DNA ligase catalyses the formation of a bond between juxtaposed 5′-phosphate (P) and 3′-hydroxyl (OH) groups on the phosphate 'backbone' of DNA.

A *transposon* is a piece of DNA, often flanked by specific repeat sequences, that can be efficiently excised from or integrated into a second DNA molecule.

without a need for compatible ends (Fig. 2.12). DNA ligase also heals 'nicks' in DNA, where *one* of the two phosphate backbone chains is broken.

Several practical considerations enter into ligating DNA fragments (Fig. 2.13). Blunt-cut vectors can close without an insert. This unwanted product of self-ligation can be reduced by dephosphorylating the vector, in which case ligation depends on the phosphate groups at the ends of the insert. Vectors with different 'sticky' ends cannot close on themselves because the overhanging ends are not compatible (they do not anneal to one another). Sticky-end ligation with different ends permits 'directional cloning', since the insert can only 'go in' one way.

Transposition—natural recombination

Transposition is a highly efficient means of generating recombinant DNA molecules. Different enzyme systems are employed by organisms ranging from bacteria to mammals but they all involve the reversible insertion of piece of foreign DNA into the genomic DNA of a host.

Nature has produced the variety of life without recourse to a laboratory. Molecular biologists have only recently begun to exploit transposition to generate recombinant DNA. The ease with which DNA pieces can be moved around threatens to take some of the art and craft out of molecular biology (Fig. 2.14).

There are two types of transposable elements:

• Class I transposons propagate by making RNA transcripts. The RNA may encode a reverse transcriptase (see below) and an integrase, which are enzymes that insert a DNA copy into the genome.

• Class II transposons are flanked by inverted repeat sequences. This transposon class may encode a *transposase*, which is an enzyme that catalyses excision and integration of the transposon.

Transposition can be an efficient means of trading large, useful pieces of DNA such as genes. However, it can also disrupt functional genes. In an important study, crosses between certain strains of fruit flies produced many mutant offspring, an effect called hybrid dysgenesis (the opposite of hybrid vigor), due to the

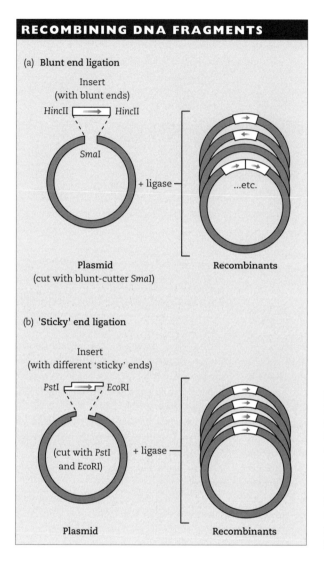

RECOMBINING DNA FRAGMENTS

(a) Blunt end ligation

Plasmid
(cut with blunt-cutter *Sma*I)

Recombinants

(b) 'Sticky' end ligation

Plasmid

Recombinants

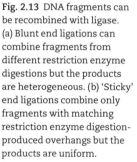

Fig. 2.13 DNA fragments can be recombined with ligase. (a) Blunt end ligations can combine fragments from different restriction enzyme digestions but the products are heterogeneous. (b) 'Sticky' end ligations combine only fragments with matching restriction enzyme digestion-produced overhangs but the products are uniform.

activation of transposition and disruption of many genes. The transposon was found to encode its own suppressor that accumulated in the cytoplasm. This transposon spread very rapidly though the worldwide population of fruit flies, providing a likely example of parasitic or 'selfish' DNA.

Class I transposons are also called retro-transposons because of their similarity to RNA viruses (retroviruses). Integrated retroviruses may account for about 1% of the human gen-ome. These are called human endogenous retroviruses (HERVs), although chimpanzees and gorillas have largely the same endogenous retroviruses, suggesting they are very old.

Human disease has also been attributed to transposition. One HERV on chromosome 7 is suspected of causing testicular cancer and other cancers. A different retroviral insertion also causes Fukuyama-type congenital muscu-lar dystrophy by interfering with the expres-sion of a secreted protein. The potential for

TRANSPOSITION: NATURE'S WAY TO RECOMBINE

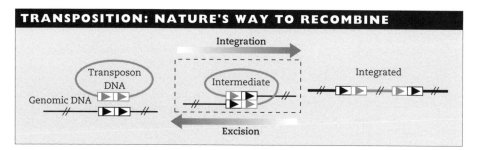

Fig. 2.14 Transposition is precise and reversible. During integration, similar or identical sequences within the transposon DNA and genomic DNA align. Both DNAs are cut within the repeat and rejoined with the other DNA. The integrated DNA that results can still be identified by the presence of flanking, direct repeat sequences. The transposon can also be excised from genomic DNA. In bacteria, these reversible reactions require only three enzymes: bacteriophage-encoded integrase (Int) and excisionase (Xis) and a bacterial protein called integration host factor (IHF).

the activation of endogenous retroviruses present in the genomes of other species is also a concern that might limit the therapeutic transplantation to humans of tissues from different animals (xenotransplantation).

DNA polymerase and nuclease—lengthening and shortening DNA

Polymerases

There are many different DNA polymerases (Pols), often several in an organism, but they have one activity in common: adding nucleotides (Fig. 2.15).

The last rule is not absolute because there *are* enzymes that polymerize DNA and work without a template strand, but these are used relatively infrequently (e.g. terminal deoxytransferase (TdT), which adds a 'tail' of nucleotides). The first two rules of DNA Pols might make you think again about how genomic

POLYMERASE RULES

- All polymerases require an end to extend; none can synthesize DNA *de novo*.
- All polymerases extend the 3'-OH end (5' → 3' polymerase); no DNA Pol adds to the 5' end.
- Nearly all polymerases make a reverse copy (the *complement*) of the template strand.

DNA is replicated. DNA Pol cannot start synthesizing DNA *de novo*, so instead replication of genomic DNA starts with RNA primers of ~10 bp length, which are first extended and then replaced with DNA by DNA Pol (see Chapter 1). Both strands are replicated as the 'replication fork' moves in one direction. Replication in the 5' → 3' direction is easy because that is the direction of DNA polymerization. In the 3' → 5' direction, small pieces of DNA (1000–2000 bp) are synthesized in the 5' → 3' direction and then ligated together.

Fig. 2.15 DNA polymerases add to the 3' end of the DNA nucleotides that match the opposite strand, the template.

POLYMERASE ADDS NUCLEOTIDES

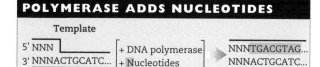

NUCLEASE ANARCHY

- Some *exo*nucleases chew from one end (5′ → 3′).
- Some *exo*nucleases chew from the other end (3′ → 5′).
- Some *endo*nucleases take a bite right out of the middle, not starting at an end.
- Some nucleases strongly prefer single-stranded DNA or RNA. This preference forms the basis of the nuclease protection assay (see p. 82).

Nucleases

Nucleases cut nucleic acids either into big pieces (*endo*nucleases) or many little pieces (*exo*nucleases). Exonucleases can be seen as undoing the work of polymerases: they depolymerize. Unlike the relatively uniform world of polymerases, however, nucleases demonstrate a wide range of abilities.

Many DNA polymerases also possess exonuclease activities. A polymerase with a 3′ → 5′ exonuclease activity (reverse of the 5′ → 3′ polymerase activity) can remove a newly added nucleotide. This activity is called 'proofreading' because it improves the fidelity of replication. DNA polymerase extends a mismatched base only slowly because it is not base paired to the template, making it appear single stranded, which gives the exonuclease activity more time to digest. A 5′ → 3′ exonuclease activity can clear the way ahead for the polymerase activity, digesting the old strand. This activity probably removes the RNA primer that initiates DNA replication.

Polymerase chain reaction (PCR)

PCR is used to amplify fragments of DNA.

This simple but incredibly powerful technique has revolutionized molecular biology and many applications have already found their way into clinical and forensic medicine. You can easily generate many copies of single DNA molecules. The recipe is simple, just add the ingredients (template, oligo primers, nucleotides, buffer, polymerase) and bake (and cool, bake again, and cool . . . , Fig. 2.16).

PCR amplifies the segment of DNA between the oligonucleotide primers, which are usually 15–25 bp long and designed to match specific sequences (5′ and 3′) flanking the segment to be amplified. Therefore, it is *usually* necessary to know these flanking sequences (although methods have been developed allowing PCR amplification of segments when only one end is known; see *PCR variations*, p. 44). DNA polymerase extends the primers after they anneal to the template, creating a duplicate, complementary strand (Fig. 2.16).

If the amplification were 100% efficient, then the number of template molecules would double every cycle ('exponential' phase amplification) and 30 cycles would produce over a thousand million-fold amplification (2^{30} = 1 073 741 824, Fig. 2.17). As great as it is, even PCR is not perfect. The latter cycles often produce linear amplification as the reagents are used up, or begin to suffer from being repeatedly cooked and cooled or simply from

DNA SYNTHESIS

Synthetic oligonucleotides (oligos) are made in the opposite direction. The chemical reaction proceeds by adding to the 5′ end, whereas the enzymatic reaction (polymerases) adds to the 3′ end.

Biology (polymerases)
$$5\text{′-NNNN-}3\text{′} \rightarrow \text{extension}$$
Chemistry (synthetic oligos)
$$\text{extension} \leftarrow 5\text{′-NNNN-}3\text{′}$$

Even with a good yield (99%) for the addition of each nucleotide, the yield of full-length oligo of 25 nucleotides (a '25mer') is only about 3 out of 4 ($0.99^{25} = 0.778$). This explains the desirability of ensuring that synthetic oligos are full length before using them in certain procedures, especially those with single base resolution (e.g. sequencing). Fortunately, the natural way to make DNA is much more efficient.

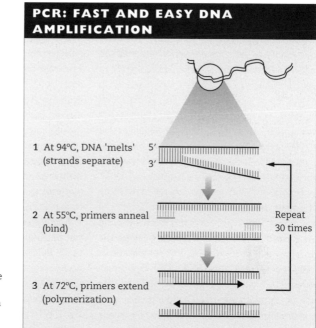

PCR: FAST AND EASY DNA AMPLIFICATION

1 At 94°C, DNA 'melts' (strands separate)

2 At 55°C, primers anneal (bind)

3 At 72°C, primers extend (polymerization)

Repeat 30 times

Fig. 2.16 'Some like it hot'. One thermal cycle in the polymerase chain reaction (PCR) is shown. Steps 1–3 double the amount of template flanked by the primers. Repeated 30 times, they yield a million-fold amplification in about 1 hour.

PHASES OF PCR AMPLIFICATION

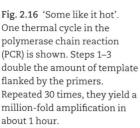

Cycle :   #1   #2   #3
Copies :1 ⟶ 2 ⟶ 4 ⟶ 8

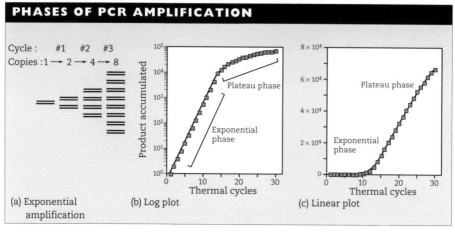

(a) Exponential amplification

(b) Log plot

(c) Linear plot

Fig. 2.17 PCR amplification of a DNA template is initially exponential. (a) Three perfectly efficient cycles are shown. To represent the million-fold amplification that can be obtained after 30 cycles, approximately 3 km would be required at this scale. Product accumulation during PCR is plotted as a function of cycle number on either a logarithmic scale (b) or a linear scale (c). PCR is often biphasic: exponential amplification in the early cycles is followed by non-exponential amplification in the later cycles, called the plateau phase. The point at which the reaction becomes non-exponential depends on the reaction conditions. Note that the significant accumulation of product during the later cycles seems to belie the name 'plateau phase'.

competition for the polymerase molecules ('plateau phase', Fig. 2.17b). Even with considerably lower overall efficiency, however, one can easily generate enough product to see on an ethidium bromide (EtBr)-stained agarose gel starting with a single copy target sequence from 1 ng of genomic DNA. This is the DNA content of approximately 1000 (nucleated) mammalian cells, which can be found in $1 \mu l$ (0.001 cc) of blood.

Legend has it that the original PCR was performed with a 'regular' (heat-sensitive) DNA polymerase (probably the so-called Klenow fragment that lacks an exonuclease activity of the intact DNA polymerase). Fresh enzyme was added for each thermal cycle because the enzyme was destroyed at the temperatures required to melt the DNA. This flaw in an otherwise beautiful procedure spurred the characterization and mass production of *heat-stable enzymes*, the first of which to be widely used was *Taq* DNA polymerase (from *Thermus aquaticus*). Several additional thermal stable DNA polymerases, RNA polymerases and DNA ligases are now available.

Accelerating PCR analysis (faster!)

The rate-limiting step in PCR is often the detection and analysis of the amplified product. For example, a portion of a viral genome may be PCR amplified in less than an hour of cycling, but analysis by gel electrophoresis requires considerable manipulation and time. Several methods have been devised to quickly determine the presence of the product. These methods require thermal cyclers that are able to detect fluorescence during cycling.

1 *Fluorogenic DNA stains.* Product accumulation can be monitored using stains that fluoresce upon binding to double-stranded DNA and do not inhibit DNA polymerization, e.g. SYBR Green I. A positive sample in such an experiment produces an upward curved line (see Fig. 2.17) while a negative sample produces a flat line. The absolute amount of template in the starting sample is calculated from a stand-

---

PCR VARIATIONS

The polymerase chain reaction (PCR) has changed molecular biology fundamentally. Here are some of the important variations of this basic reaction.

'Hot Start' is the most generally applicable variation. A critical reaction component is withheld until the reaction is hot (> 60°C), when the component is added and the reaction starts. This means that the stringency of the primer annealing is high when the DNA polymerase is allowed to extend the primer, greatly increasing the specificity. This protocol also illustrates the distinction between specificity of amplification, which is most stringent at high temperatures, and the amount of amplification, which may be greater at lower temperatures.

'Touchdown' PCR tries for the best of both worlds, using a high annealing temperature at the beginning of cycling to enforce specificity and then gradually lowering the temperature to encourage amplification.

'Long and Accurate' PCR (LA-PCR) was invented to overcome the limitations of conventional Taq polymerase, which does not work well for large templates (> 2 kb) because this relatively error-prone enzyme introduces mutations that accumulate and block efficient extension and product formation. This is overcome by the addition of small amounts of a proofreading polymerase that corrects the errors, allowing the completion of nascent chains. With this small modification and longer extension times (roughly 1 minute per kb), products of > 10 kb can be efficiently amplified.

Two methods allow templates whose sequence is known only at one end to be PCR amplified. In 'anchored' PCR the unknown end is extended with dCTPs and the template-independent DNA polymerase TdT (see *Polymerases*). An oligo dG is annealed to the tail and used as the 'other' primer. Alternatively, in 'ligation-mediated' PCR, the unknown end is ligated to a double-stranded oligonucleotide, to which a matching primer is annealed.

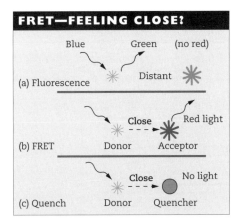

FRET—FEELING CLOSE?

(a) Fluorescence

Blue   Green   (no red)

Distant

(b) FRET

Close   Red light

Donor   Acceptor

(c) Quench

Close   No light

Donor   Quencher

Fig. 2.18 The phenomenon called fluorescence resonance energy transfer (FRET) underlies many new analyses. (a) fluorescence occurs when light energy at a certain frequency excites a compound, called a fluor, which then relaxes by emitting light at a second frequency. Here, incident blue light excites and green light is emitted. A second fluor is not excited by blue light. (b) When different fluors are close enough (approximately 5 nm, or two times the width of a double-stranded DNA helix), an excited donor fluor can transfer energy without light emission directly to a second acceptor fluor. The second fluor emits light at a different frequency, here red. (c) A special acceptor called a quencher efficiently absorbs the fluorescence of the first fluor but does not itself fluoresce.

ard curve generated using known amounts of template.

2 *Fluorescence resonance energy transfer (FRET)* is a very sensitive measure of the distance between two different molecules (Fig. 2.18). This phenomenon has been applied to measuring specific PCR products (Fig. 2.19). In contrast to the use of fluorogenic stain, specific FRET probes permit the detection of multiple templates amplified simultaneously in one sample, a process known as multiplexing.

Two FRET adaptations are widely used for continuous 'real-time' measurement. One known as Molecular Beacons uses a probe that forms a hairpin loop, juxtaposing the donor and quencher (Fig. 2.19a). At annealing temperatures, the 5–7 nucleotide 'arms' can form

the stem, or the loop of 10–40 nucleotides can bind to the target sequence, resulting in fluorescence. Note that this probe melts off the target sequence at polymerizing temperature so Taq extension is not blocked. A second assay called TaqMan ('Tack man') is named after the old video game character, Pac-Man, that eats everything in its path (Fig. 2.19b). The assay depends on the $3' \rightarrow 5'$ exonuclease activity of Taq, which normally clears a path ahead of the $5' \rightarrow 3'$ polymerase activity. Single-stranded probes annealed to the template are degraded by Taq, freeing the fluorescent reporter from the quencher.

Fluorescent (and bioluminescent) labels are quickly displacing radioactivity in research and clinical laboratories. Several factors contribute to this trend. Highly sensitive cameras and low-power lasers have become inexpensive. The chemistries for labelling nucleic acids and proteins have been simplified. Meanwhile, costs of using radioactivity, especially safety and disposal, have increased. Multiple fluorescent or bioluminescent probes can also be used simultaneously, an approach called multiplexing, because the signals can be resolved based on their different wavelengths (spectra). These trends make for lighter work.

Isothermal nucleic acid amplification— some like it cooler . . .

Future amplification systems may be non-thermal cycling (isothermal). Room-temperature or 'warm' amplification/detection systems may have particular application in clinical testing, where time is critical and thoroughly tested reagent kits can be prepared for specific assays. For example, the amplification of pathogen-specific DNA or RNA may allow the rapid identification of infections or monitoring of a patient's response to treatment. These three systems illustrate the promise of isothermal amplification.

• The self-sustained synthesis reaction (3SR, also called nucleic acid synthesis-based amplification, NASBA) is a combination of reactions modelled on retrovirus replication. An RNA template is *reverse transcribed* into DNA, which

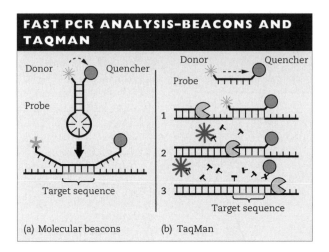

FAST PCR ANALYSIS–BEACONS AND TAQMAN

(a) Molecular beacons   (b) TaqMan

Fig. 2.19 Fluorogenic assays accelerate PCR analysis. (a) With molecular beacons, a donor fluor is fixed to the 5′ end of an oligonucleotide and a quencher is fixed to the 3′ end. The complementary ends form a short stem in a hairpin loop structure. The sequence in the middle of the probe anneals to the target sequence, disrupting the loop and separating the quencher from the donor. (b) With TaqMan, the donor fluor and quencher are fixed to the opposite ends of the probe oligonucleotide, which anneals to the target sequence. During PCR, the exonuclease activity of Taq clears the path ahead of the polymerase activity by degrading the probe oligo, separating the fluor from the quencher.

is then *transcribed*, generating more RNAs that are *reverse transcribed* and so on. Transcription and reverse transcription reactions proceed simultaneously within the test tube, establishing a massively parallel system that can produce a 10 thousand million-fold (10^{10}) amplification in 90 minutes.

• Qβ-replicase is a novel RNA polymerase derived from a bacteriophage that can produce 100 million-fold (10^8) amplification in 15 minutes. The template for Qβ-replicase is an RNA that is folded into a particular shape. Both 3SR and Qβ-replicase amplify RNA directly, which can be an advantage over conventional PCR. However, the amplified products are also RNAs, which are more difficult to analyse.

• Rolling circle amplification (RCA) is modelled on the replication of circular DNAs such as the genomes of bacteria and some viruses. A primer oligonucleotide, usually tethered to a location by a variety of means, is annealed to a circular template and extended by polymerase. Unlike the amplifications described above, which occur in solution, RCA has the unique attribute of being easily localized. This is useful for *in situ* analyses, such as histology, and microarray probes (see Chapter 3).

Refined, such methods might make the coffee maker the only thermal cycler in the laboratory or clinic.

RNA polymerase and reverse transcriptase—making RNA from DNA and vice versa

RNA polymerase

RNA polymerases make RNA from a DNA template (transcription).

There are three RNA polymerases (RNA Pols) in mammals that are responsible for reading the DNA code and generating matching (complementary) RNA, which either does the real work itself or is translated into protein (Fig. 2.20).

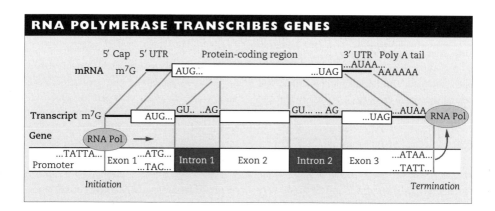

RNA POLYMERASE TRANSCRIBES GENES

Fig. 2.20 Genes are transcribed by RNA polymerase (RNA Pol). Transcription initiates when RNA polymerase recognizes specific nucleotide sequences, usually located in the gene promoter. Nucleotide sequences that signal important transcription and processing steps are shown.

- RNA Pol I transcribes the rRNA genes.
- RNA Pol II transcribes the protein-coding genes, making mRNA.
- RNA Pol III transcribes the tRNA genes.

Pol II is the most intensively studied because of its role in gene and protein expression. Gene expression is often regulated by the rate of transcription, which is largely controlled by the binding of RNA Pol II to the gene promoter. Since RNA Pol II must transcribe many different genes, it is helped to identify exactly which gene should be transcribed and when by gene-specific proteins. These proteins bind to sequences in the gene, called enhancers or silencers, that act to increase or decrease the frequency of transcription. Additional proteins help RNA Pol II to find exactly the correct start (initiation) and end (termination).

In front of the gene is the promoter, which binds RNA polymerase and is largely respons-ible for regulating transcription (Fig. 2.20). The gene contains exons, which encode the mat-ure mRNA, and introns, which interrupt the protein-coding region of the gene and primary transcript but are spliced out during mRNA maturation. Introns start with GU (splice

donor) and end with AG (splice acceptor). The rate of splicing can influence gene expression. Some exons can be skipped, which is called alternative splicing and can dramatically change the function of the encoded protein. The protein-coding region is flanked by 5' and 3' untranslated regions (UTRs) that regulate mRNA translation and stability. The protein-coding sequence of the transcript starts with the triplet nucleic acid codon AUG, which encodes the amino acid methionine, and ends with one of the three codons that does not

READING THE HELICAL DNA TEMPLATE

It is not known exactly how RNA polymerase manages to read the helical DNA template, analogous to reading an inscription circling round a column, without getting the ever lengthening RNA transcript hopelessly tangled. It is likely that the DNA is nicked and then rotates around the (other) single strand beneath the RNA polymerase. One reason this is thought to be true is because in bacteria the RNA message is already being translated before transcription is complete and it seems improbable that the whole RNA polymerase–mRNA–ribosome complex could spin around the DNA. Although RNA polymerase is fast (bacterial RNA polymerase adds 60 nucleotides/second), at this rate it takes nearly an hour to transcribe the 186 000-bp gene encoding the human clotting factor VII.

encode an amino acid, either UAA, UAG, or UGA. The 7-methyl guanosine (m^7G) structure called a 'cap' is added to the mRNA almost immediately upon transcription initiation, whereas the poly(A) tail is added following the signal AAUAAA at the end of the mRNA sequence.

Bacteriophage polymerases —simply useful

Relatively simple RNA polymerases from the bacteriophages named T7 and SP6 are very useful for making large amounts of a given transcript. These are small, single-polypeptide enzymes that have been cloned and are widely available at low cost and high activity. They initiate transcription at short (~12 bp) promoters. To generate RNA transcripts for probes or translation templates, the gene of interest can be placed 'downstream' (3') of the appropriate promoter. Just add ribonucleotides (rNTPs) and RNA polymerase and incubate.

Reverse transcriptase

Reverse transcriptase (RT) makes complementary DNA from an RNA template.

In the beginning, the word was that genetic information could go in only one direction, from DNA to RNA to protein. The dogma was shaken when it was found that viruses with an RNA genome (retroviruses) replicate through a DNA intermediate. The descriptive name *reverse transcription* was given to this activity, and the responsible enzymes are called RT (Fig. 2.21).

The ability to reverse transcribe mRNA into cDNA helps in gene cloning and recombinant protein production because the introns are eliminated, often greatly reducing the size of the DNA to be cloned and expressed. Also, recombinant proteins encoded by cDNA can be produced in bacteria, which do not have introns and do not have the splicing mechanisms to remove introns. Using cDNA, one can clone and analyse the protein-coding part of a gene and then proceed directly to producing the protein in large quantities (see *cDNA cloning* and *Recombinant proteins*, Chapter 3).

General methods

Blotting

Blotting is a descriptive term for the *transfer of molecules out of a gel and onto a filter membrane by wicking action* (Fig. 2.22). The term is now used for electro- or vacuum transfers, and even for simply binding to filters molecules that were not resolved on a gel ('dot blots'). Blotting was developed to make the nucleic acids resolved on a gel more accessible to subsequent manipulation, such as identification by hybridization (see next section).

In a Southern blot, DNA is separated by movement through a non-denaturing gel, then denatured with sodium hydroxide and blotted. The blot is then probed with either labelled DNA or RNA. The gel may also be a denaturing urea/polyacrylamide gel, in which case denaturation prior to transfer is not necessary. The Southern blot is named after its originator, Dr Edwin Southern.

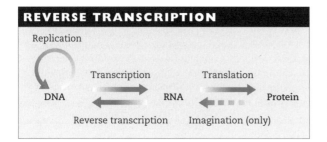

Fig. 2.21 The enzyme reverse transcriptase generates complementary DNA from RNA. Reverse translation, if it were ever observed, could not be precise due to the degeneracy of the genetic code (nearly every amino acid can be encoded by two or more triplet nucleotide codons).

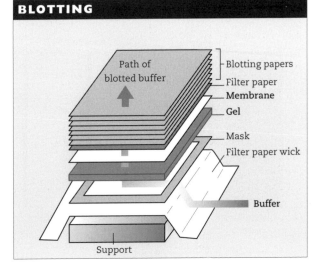

BLOTTING

Fig. 2.22 Blotting carries nucleic acids out of gels and onto membranes. The stack of filter papers, gel, membrane and blotting paper is held out of the buffer bath by the support. The blotting papers absorb buffer and wicking action (absorption) pulls the buffer up through the gel, carrying the nucleic acids along, and then through the membrane, to which the nucleic acid binds. The mask ensures that the buffer goes through the gel rather than around it.

In a Northern blot, RNA is separated by movement through an agarose gel containing a denaturing agent (formamide/formaldehyde) and blotted. The blot is then probed with labelled DNA or RNA. The Northern blot was named whimsically *after* the Southern blot.

In a Western blot, proteins are separated by movement through a gel containing a denaturing detergent (sodium dodecyl sulphate (SDS)/polyacrylamide gel), and then blotted and detected with antibodies. To complete the naming, DNA-binding proteins are detected in a South-western blot and RNA-binding proteins are detected in a North-western blot. In these assays, proteins are separated and then probed with nucleic acids. The future directions in blotting techniques seem clear.

Hybridization and annealing

Hybridization is the formation of base pairs between nucleic acids. The term was originally restricted to the formation of *hybrid* double-stranded molecules, as in a Northern blot where DNA/RNA hybrid molecules are formed. Typically, a mixture of nucleic acids is resolved on a gel, blotted onto a nitrocellulose or nylon membrane, and the blot is hybridized with a labelled (easily detectable) piece of DNA or RNA called the probe (Fig. 2.23). The

probe sticks to its complementary strand (hybridizes), the blot is washed to remove unbound and non-specifically bound probe and the remaining probe is then detected. The method of detection depends on how the probe was labelled. Probes are often labelled with radioactive nucleotides and the probe is detected by autoradiography (self-exposure on film).

The longer the length of hybridized strands, the stronger the binding (up to about 100 bp). By using more or less stringent conditions to wash away unbound and weakly bound probe, it is possible to determine how well the probe is bound to the blotted target nucleic acid (Table 2.4). High temperature and the organic solvent formamide tend to make the hybridized strands come apart, whereas high salt concentration and aqueous solutions stabilize the hybrid by shielding the negative phosphate charges.

A blot is hybridized at *high* stringency to detect only the nucleic acids that are *closely related or identical* to the probe. A blot is probed (hybridized and washed) at *low* stringency to detect more *distantly related* sequences. This might be done to identify additional members of a multigene family or homologous genes in other species.

BLOT AND HYBRIDIZE

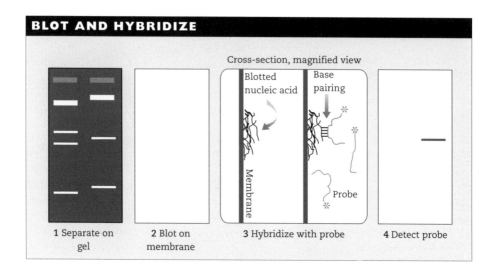

1 Separate on gel   2 Blot on membrane   3 Hybridize with probe   4 Detect probe

Fig. 2.23 Specific sequences can be detected in a mixture of nucleic acids by separating them on a gel, blotting, and hybridizing with a sequence-specific probe. The method of detection depends on the type of label on the probe. Typically, the probe is radioactively labelled and detected on photographic film (autoradiography).

Synthetic oligonucleotides (oligos) may be used in detecting blotted nucleotides. Base pairing with the complementary nucleic acid is also called *annealing*, a term that is used especially often for oligos. Hybridization protocols must be specifically adapted to oligos because the shorter probes form hybrids with lower stability. There are also advantages of using oligos as probes. They are easy to make (just fax the sequence to your favourite biotech company), easy to label, and strand specific. For example, a complementary oligo would be ideal to detect messenger RNA (mRNA) or perhaps block gene expression (see *Antisense oligonucleotides*, Chapter 3).

The strength of DNA–DNA bonds can be calculated from the nucleotide sequences. As would be expected from the number of bonds formed, the A-T pairs are approximately two-thirds as strong as G-C pairs. However, the overall stability of the duplex is not just a sum of these bonds. The stability of each nucleotide pair is strongly influenced by the neighbouring nucleotide pairs. Fortunately, all 10 of the possible nearest neighbour interactions have been measured, permitting the stability of any duplex to be accurately predicted from the sequence.

CONDITIONS REGULATE CROSS HYBRIDIZATION

Hybridize/wash conditions	Low stringency	High stringency
Temperature	Low	High
Formamide concentration	Low	High
Salt concentration	High	Low
Use for detecting genes that are	Similar	*versus* Identical

Table 2.4 The stringency of blot hybridization and washing conditions can be modified to control the extent of cross hybridization between the probe and different genes.

Transfection and transformation —selection and screening

Transfection and transformation are ways of putting genes into cells. Selection and screening are ways of finding the cells that received the genes.

Two different names are given to the process of putting genes back into cells. Bacterial cells are said to be *transformed* because in a classic experiment non-pathogenic bacteria were made pathogenic by addition of the 'transforming principle', i.e. DNA. Mammalian cells are *transfected* because the transfer of genes is similar to viral infection. Both cell types spontaneously pick up DNA, but the efficiency is very low. Numerous transfection techniques have been developed to increase the efficiency of uptake, such as the following.
• Calcium phosphate precipitation—DNA forms aggregates that precipitate and are endocytosed by the cells.
• DEAE-dextran—this cationic gel and DNA form large aggregates, which are endocytosed.
• Cationic liposomes—coat the (anionic) DNA in lipid so that it passes more readily through the cell membrane.
• 'Biolistics'—DNA is coated onto gold particles that are shot into the cells or tissues.
• Electroporation—creates transient DNA-permeable holes in the cell membrane by a high-voltage shock.
• Infection ('transduction')—genes are 'packaged' into infectious viral particles.

Despite these advances, transfection of mammalian cells often results in only a small fraction of the cells receiving DNA into their nucleus. This DNA is typically not replicated and rapidly diluted or lost from the nucleus upon cell division. A few cells become stable transfectants by incorporating the transfected DNA into their chromosomes. Many experiments are designed to find out what you want to know *before* the DNA is lost from the cell. These are called *transient transfections* (or simply transients) because they last only a few days. Transients are good for testing many different DNA constructs and in situations where the recipient cells cannot be cultured for extended times, which is often true for normal cells. Stable transfections are easier to characterize in depth and they can provide a more physiological setting for testing the response of DNA fragments that control gene activity (see *Transcription regulation*, Fig. 2.27).

With the low efficiency of transformation and transfection, the second problem is to identify the cells that have taken up DNA. This is accomplished by either *screening* or *selecting* positive clones, or by a combination. An example of selection is when bacteria are transformed with a plasmid containing a gene that confers antibiotic resistance. The few cells that take up the plasmid and express the gene will be able to grow in medium containing the antibiotic, e.g. ampicillin, while the other cells will not (Fig. 2.24). Similarly, stable mammalian cells transfected with a gene for resistance to a toxin can be selected in a toxin-containing medium. G418 or hygromycin B are examples of these toxins.

Alternatively, the expression of a plasmid-encoded enzyme in the cell might be easy to detect even though it does not change the growth characteristics or confer any resistance. This is *screening* for expression. A commonly used enzyme is β-galactosidase (β-gal), whose activity can be assayed with chromogenic substrates that either remain soluble or precipitate. For example, the β-gal-catalysed conversion of a colourless compound called Xgal (the real name is very long) to a blue precipitate allows the identification of β-gal$^+$ bacteria or animal cells (Fig. 2.25).

Many experiments call for a combination of selection and screening. The plasmids used in cloning genes usually confer resistance to antibiotics (selection) and contain a β-gal gene that is disrupted by the recombinant genes (screening, Fig. 2.25). The clones that contain recombinant DNA have an interrupted *lacZ′* gene, do not make β-gal and do not turn blue when plated on Xgal. Only these 'white' clones are picked and further tested to determine

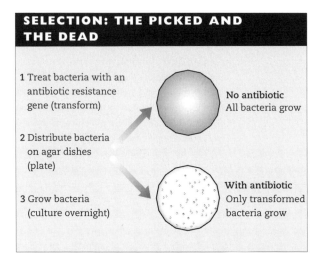

SELECTION: THE PICKED AND THE DEAD

1 Treat bacteria with an antibiotic resistance gene (transform)

No antibiotic
All bacteria grow

2 Distribute bacteria on agar dishes (plate)

With antibiotic
Only transformed bacteria grow

3 Grow bacteria (culture overnight)

Fig. 2.24 Antibiotics select for transformed bacteria. Bacteria that pick up the DNA containing the ampicillin resistance gene are able to grow on agar containing ampicillin (antibiotic resistance). The transforming DNA usually includes additional genes that are not so easily selected.

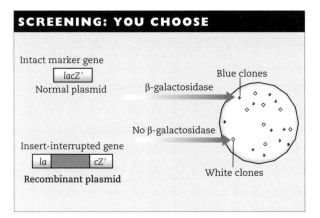

SCREENING: YOU CHOOSE

Intact marker gene
lacZ′
Normal plasmid

β-galactosidase

Blue clones

No β-galactosidase

Insert-interrupted gene
la   cZ′
Recombinant plasmid

White clones

Fig. 2.25 Blue/white screening for bacteria containing normal and recombinant lacZ′ marker genes. The lacZ′ gene encodes a critical portion of the enzyme β-galactosidase (β-gal). When cultured in the presence of Xgal (a chromogenic substrate of β-gal) and an inducer of β-gal expression, bacteria that synthesize β-gal can be found because they turn blue. Screening is usually combined with simultaneous selection for antibiotic resistance.

whether the insert is correct. Note that these subsequent tests are often also a form of screening, e.g. looking for particular restriction enzyme sites, but they are much more difficult and slower. A powerful early screen saves time; just how much time is saved depends on the frequency of 'positive' clones.

Another common combination of selection and screening occurs when making monoclonal antibodies in mammalian cells (see *Monoclonal antibodies*, Chapter 4). Hybridoma cell lines are cell fusions (hybrids) that secrete monoclonal antibodies. They are generated when an antibody-secreting normal (mortal) cell is fused *in vitro* with an immortalized cell line that is mutant in the *hypoxanthine guanine phosphoribosyl transferase* (HGPRT) gene. (This gene is encoded on the X chromosome and there is only one active copy per cell.) The hybrids receive a functional HGPRT gene from the normal cell and can thus grow in a medium that selects for HGPRT function, whilst the otherwise immortal cells are killed in this medium. Only after the hybridoma cell lines are selected for growth are they then screened for antibody secretion.

Protein–protein interactions

DNA and RNA may be glamorous, but proteins probably perform most of the cellular housekeeping. How can we apply our facility with nucleic acids to helping understand how proteins interact? In the benighted, biochemical past, you would have had to purify the protein or generate an antibody to your protein, which you would have used to literally and physically pull out interacting proteins. You would have then tried to identify these interacting proteins by testing a number of informed guesses. The modern way is to let microbes do (some of) the work.

Hybrids, fusions, chimeras and tags

Proteins are composed of smaller units, called domains, that perform particular functions. The activity of a protein is the sum of these functions. Domains are generally formed by discrete, non-overlapping lengths of *contiguous* amino acids. This arrangement also allows functions to be more easily duplicated or swapped between proteins, greatly accelerating the evolution of new proteins and protein functions. Moreover, in eukaryotes, domains are typically encoded within single exons, making the exchanges even easier. These observations were key to integrating our understanding of how proteins function and evolve.

The domain structure of proteins makes it easier for you, as well as nature, to add or delete particular functions. An easily detected domain is often called a 'tag' and when two existing proteins are put together the new proteins are called fusions, hybrids or chimeras. A few examples of these proteins are described below.

Two-hybrid screening

Two-hybrid screening is a powerful way to find new interacting proteins and clone the genes encoding them (Fig. 2.26a). One measure of a technique's success is the number of variations it spawns. With the variation called one-hybrid screening, you can clone different transcription activator domains or DNA-binding domains (the two domains at the ends of the two-hybrid system). Reverse two-hybrid allows you to clone proteins that *disrupt* interactions between two proteins.

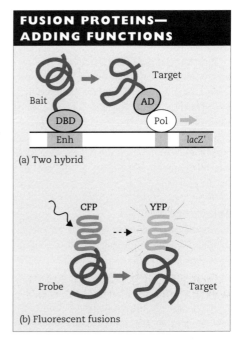

FUSION PROTEINS— ADDING FUNCTIONS

(a) Two hybrid

(b) Fluorescent fusions

Fig. 2.26 Fusion proteins help elucidate pathways of protein interactions. (a) The two-hybrid screen finds proteins that interact with a known protein called the bait. The interaction between the bait and the new target protein brings their fused domains together: the transcription-activating domain (AD) and the DNA-binding domain (DBD). This increases transcription of the *lacZ'* gene, which can be screened by colour (see Fig. 2.25). (b) Fluorescent fusion proteins are excellent for determining the cellular location of a protein. Proteins can be tracked to the nucleus, the Golgi, etc. Two proteins that are thought to interact might be colocalized by microscopy. A more precise proximity measurement can be made using fluorescent fusion proteins as probes in FRET (see Fig. 2.18). Efficient FRET occurs only when the donor and acceptor fluors are within 5 nm, which is about two to three times the width of the DNA helix. CFP, YFP; cyan or yellow fluorescent protein.

Fluorescent fusion proteins

Green fluorescent protein (GFP), just as it sounds, is a protein that fluoresces green. The original GFP was purified from a jellyfish and is excitable with ultraviolet light. Useful variants have been created that are structurally similar but are excited with visible light ('enhanced' or eGFP) or fluoresce blue or yellow or cyan (B/Y/CFP).

Surprisingly, fusing the relatively large fluorescent domain with a protein does not usually change its behaviour. This allows a fusion protein, which is easily located within in living cells, to act as a marker for the endogenous protein. The fluorescent fusion proteins can also be used to measure the distance between two proteins by FRET (Fig. 2.26b; see also Fig. 2.18).

Epitope tag

Antibodies are useful for getting a 'handle' on protein, in order to purify it or follow where it goes. The portion of the protein (or carbohydrate, or anything) that is bound by an antibody is called an epitope. Instead of trying to raise a strong, specific antiserum against every new protein, you can tag your protein with an epitope for which strong antisera are already available.

Examples of epitope tags include:
• haemagglutinin (HA), which is a short peptide derived from the influenza protein; and
• myc, which is a portion of the oncogene.
These tags are similar but are not typically used with antibodies:
• 6 × histidine (His) tag is six amino acids in a row and bound by nickel;
• glutathione-S-transferase (GST) tag is popular for purification and is easily removed.

Biochemistry

The availability of many high quality reagents has taken some of the onus from this standard approach to analysing signalling pathways. The reversible addition of a phosphate group (PO_4) is a key activity in intracellular signalling. Phosphorylation pathways can be analysed with antibodies that are specific for the form of protein containing phosphate. For example, a platelet-derived growth factor (PDGF) acts by binding to a specific cell surface receptor, triggering a series of phosphorylations of a whole host of cellular proteins. The roles of different kinases (enzymes that phosphorylate) can be analysed with inhibitor compounds that are selective for particular phosphorylation steps.

Nucleic acid–protein interactions

Overview

Gene expression is regulated by proteins that act as messengers, bringing the news of the world to the nucleus. The proteins activate or repress gene expression by recognizing specific DNA sequences, called enhancers or silencers, near the gene (Fig. 2.27). Enhancers bind proteins called activators, which interact with and stabilize transcription initiation complexes and increase the rate of transcription. Silencers bind repressors, which destabilize initiation complexes and decrease the rate of transcription.

Several methods of analysing regulatory sequences are described here. An enhancer or silencer DNA sequence can be identified in a reporter gene assay. The proteins binding to the DNA sequence can be analysed in the electrophoretic mobility shift assay (EMSA) or footprinting binding assays. Finally, binding factors that are potential transcription factors can be functionally tested in the reporter gene assay.

Reporter gene assay

Reporter genes are used to locate ('map') DNA sequences that regulate transcription.

Reporter genes are used to test whether pieces of DNA are involved in regulating the expression of the gene of interest. For example, a putative enhancer might be tested by placing a copy near a reporter gene (Fig. 2.28). If the piece of DNA increases expression of the reporter gene (i.e. it acts as an enhancer for the reporter gene) then it is assumed to function also as an enhancer for the original gene. Similarly, a sequence that is thought to stabilize mRNA might be tested by inserting

Fig. 2.27 Constitutive transcription is the basal rate of gene transcription. Different genes are transcribed constitutively at different rates. An enhancer is a DNA sequence that binds protein activators and increases transcription of a specific gene. A silencer is a DNA sequence that binds repressors and decreases transcription of a specific gene. When transcription increases, DNA polymerases initiate transcription more often but they move down the gene (transcribe) at the same speed.

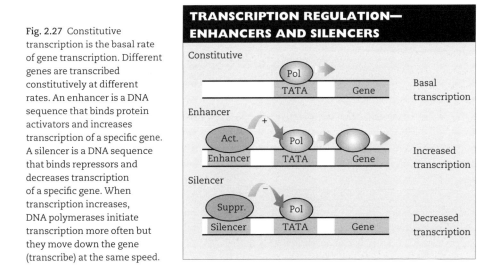

TRANSCRIPTION REGULATION— ENHANCERS AND SILENCERS

it into the 3′ UTR of a reporter gene and measuring its effect on the stability of the reporter mRNA. The important function of reporter genes is that they provide a test for an isolated part of a gene, so whatever effect is observed, it is probably caused by the fragment. However, some genetic elements probably only function in certain contexts, such as when they are together with many other elements, so the interpretation of reporter gene results can be difficult.

The *useful* aspect of reporter genes is that their products are easy to measure (Table 2.5). Since the gene of interest is replaced by something else, it might as well be replaced by something with an easily assayed gene product.

If the sequence of a regulatory element identified in a reporter gene assay resembles the sequence recognized by a previously characterized DNA-binding protein, then that protein is a good candidate for regulating the reporter gene. The reporter gene assay can be reversed to test directly the putative transcription factor, instead of their binding site. A reporter gene under control of the regulatory DNA element is cotransfected along with an expression vector that produces the candidate transcription factor. If the transcription factor binds to the regulatory element and

modulates transcription (as measured in the reporter gene assay), then the factor is likely to regulate the gene through binding to the DNA sequence.

Electrophoretic mobility shift assay (EMSA)—'gel shift'

> The EMSA is used to detect specific DNA-binding proteins. These proteins are potential regulators of gene expression.

DNA sequences act as enhancers or repressors by binding specific proteins. These proteins can be characterized in an electrophoretic mobility shift assay (EMSA) in which fragments of the gene are labelled and incubated with proteins extracted from the nucleus (Fig. 2.29).

A modified form of the EMSA can identify the proteins binding to DNA sequences. An antibody that is specific for a known protein is added to the DNA binding mix (Fig. 2.29, step 1). The complex does not change if the antibody does not bind the protein. If the antibody binds to the protein, however, then either the formation of the DNA–protein complex is blocked or a larger complex with decreased mobility is formed ('supershifted').

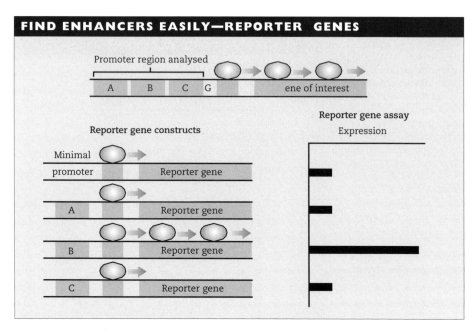

FIND ENHANCERS EASILY—REPORTER GENES

Promoter region analysed

A B C G

ene of interest

Reporter gene assay

Reporter gene constructs

Expression

Minimal

promoter   Reporter gene

A   Reporter gene

B   Reporter gene

C   Reporter gene

Fig. 2.28 Reporter gene assay of enhancer function in transfected cells. The minimal promoter (a TATA box and transcription initiation site) is inactive when transfected into a suitable recipient cell, so the reporter gene is not expressed and no product accumulates. Fragments of the promoter of the gene of interest are placed in front of the inactive, minimal promoter, and these constructs are tested (fragments A, B and C). The expression of the reporter gene is greatly increased by the B region, suggesting that this fragment of the promoter contains an enhancer.

Table 2.5 Comparison of common reporter genes.

REPORTER GENES AND THEIR PRODUCTS

Reporter gene	Assay method	Advantages
Chloramphenicol acetyl transferase (CAT)	Radiochemical enzyme assay	Sensitive; many constructs already exist because it is *the old standard*
β-Galactosidase	Chromogenic enzyme assay	Insensitive but cheap and safe; allows quantification of transfection efficiency
Luciferase (luc)	Luminescence (light production)	Very sensitive; near-zero background in mammalian cells because it is a firefly gene
Human growth hormone (hGH)	Radioimmunoassay	Sensitive and a secreted product, so the medium is tested without lysing the cells
Green fluorescent protein (GFP)	Fluorescence microscopy, etc.	Sensitive, quantitative, non-destructive and, best of all, very easy!

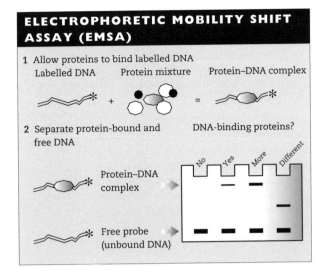

ELECTROPHORETIC MOBILITY SHIFT ASSAY (EMSA)

1 Allow proteins to bind labelled DNA

Labelled DNA   Protein mixture   Protein–DNA complex

2 Separate protein-bound and free DNA

DNA-binding proteins?

Protein–DNA complex

No   Yes   More   Different

Free probe (unbound DNA)

Fig. 2.29 The EMSA, also known as 'gel shift' assay, detects DNA-binding proteins. The DNA bound to protein moves more slowly than the free DNA through the gel (its mobility is reduced).

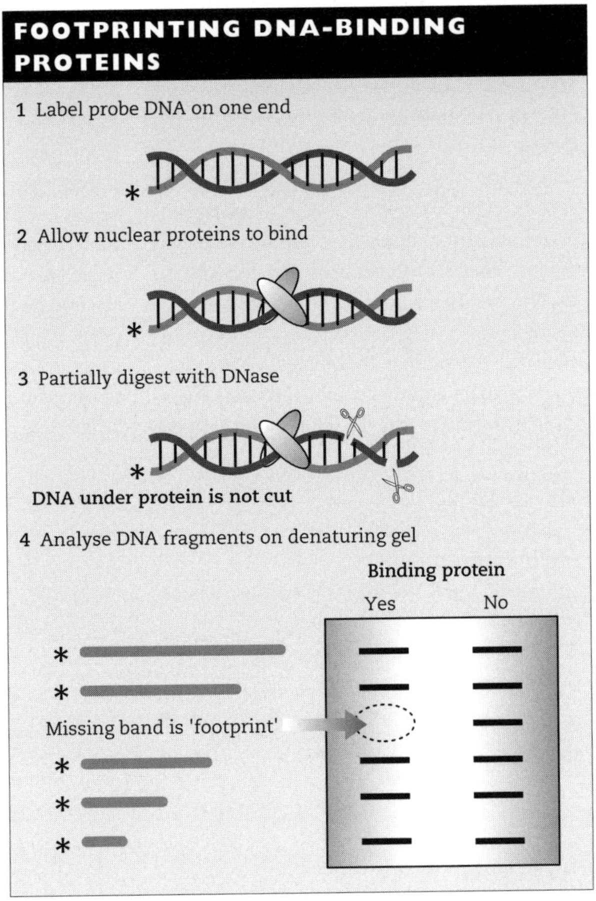

FOOTPRINTING DNA-BINDING PROTEINS

1 Label probe DNA on one end

2 Allow nuclear proteins to bind

3 Partially digest with DNase

DNA under protein is not cut

4 Analyse DNA fragments on denaturing gel

Binding protein

Yes   No

Missing band is 'footprint'

Fig. 2.30 Proteins binding to a regulatory DNA sequence leave a 'footprint' upon treatment with DNase. The DNA region that is tested is known to have a function, such as an enhancer. Without the protective DNA-binding proteins, all of the DNA would be digested. DNase I can cut every unprotected phosphodiester bond between nucleotides, so the real gel would contain very many bands.

Footprinting

Footprinting is used to detect and finely map specific DNA-binding proteins. These proteins are potential regulators of gene expression.

Footprinting is another way to analyse DNA-binding proteins. Footprinting is a nuclease protection assay in which the protector is a protein rather than an annealed oligonucleotide (Fig. 2.30).

The footprinting assay reveals additional detail about the DNA–protein interaction, information that is not easily obtained from the EMSA.

Footprinting provides:
• Resolution of the *contact points* between the protein and DNA at the nucleotide level. DNase is excluded from areas of close contact (yielding the footprint), so areas that are digested are unlikely to be involved in the binding.
• Information about the *DNA structure* in the DNA–protein complex. DNase I *hypersensitive* sites are often observed alongside protected regions. Hypersensitive sites are thought to result from a bend in the DNA induced by protein binding.

Finally, a modified footprinting procedure can determine whether a DNA–protein interaction observed *in vitro* occurs *in vivo*, inside the

EMSA OR FOOTPRINTING?

DNA-binding proteins are detected in both the DNase footprinting assay and the EMSA but there is an important difference between these assays. A shifted band is seen in the EMSA even if only a small fraction of the probe DNA is bound. In contrast, a large fraction of the probe DNA in the footprint assay must be bound and protected to be able to detect a missing band. This practical consideration may be one reason why the EMSA is used more often although footprinting can be more informative.

cell. This is important because the relatively large amounts of proteins and DNA that are used *in vitro* can produce misleading, artefactual binding. DNase I cannot be used in this assay because it does not pass through cellular membranes. Instead, chemicals such as dimethylsulphate (DMS) are used because they are membrane permeable and react with DNA to form derivatives of nucleotides, as in DNA sequencing by the Maxam–Gilbert method. Living cells are treated briefly with DMS and then the genomic DNA is prepared. The DNA is cleaved at the derivatized nucleotides and the fragments are separated on a gel. The footprint, which is formed when binding proteins exclude DMS from reacting with the DNA, can be detected on a Southern blot or, for very little DNA, after PCR amplification.

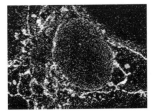

Understanding Genetics

Genes encode the proteins and the RNAs that comprise the structural components of the organism, or act as enzymes to direct the formation of these components, such as lipids and carbohydrates. Here we will review how genes are inherited, how they can change (mutate), how these changes can influence life. Finding mutations and determining how they affect life are important applications of current technology. Correcting or compensating for mutations is the aim of gene therapy.

Historical primer: genetics in a pea pod

Gregor Mendel (1860) determined the basic laws of inheritance by following seven traits of garden peas though several generations. He concluded that each pea contains two particles (genes) that encode each trait and that each offspring inherits, independent of the other genes, one version of each particle (allele) from each parent. His insight was enabled by two simplifications. First, he followed traits with simple dominant or recessive expression patterns, such as red or white flower colour. Second, he followed traits encoded by genes that are not linked.

The first to note that Mendel's rules apply to certain human traits and diseases was Archibald Garrod (1900). W. S. Sutton (1900) postulated that genes are carried on structures called chromosomes ('coloured bodies'), so called because they can be stained and observed by light microscopy (see also Chapter 1). The consequences of chromosomes, which link genes together, and variable expression, which produces intermediate or mixed traits, were elucidated in peas and fruit flies by William Bateson, R. C. Punnett and T. H. Morgan (1910).

Oswald Avery (1940) showed that genes are made of DNA. The DNA sequences are linked end to end, forming enormously long molecules that are packaged with specialized proteins into chromosomes. James Watson and Francis Crick (1950) determined the double helical structure of DNA, which immediately suggested mechanisms for replication. Barbara McClintock (1950) revolutionized genetics by showing in corn that the genome is dynamic and that genes and whole chromosomal regions can move. Increasing complexity should not obscure the amazing truth that the genetic mechanisms of inheritance employed by plants and animals are essentially identical.

Basic cellular functions are often performed by proteins that are encoded by ancient and highly conserved genes. For example, histone 2A proteins in a *garden pea* and a *human* are identical at 93 out of 118 amino acids.

Transmitting genes: inheritance

Human somatic cells (any cell other than an egg or sperm) are said to have 23 pairs of chromosomes (although the X–Y sex chromosomes do not pair). Each chromosome has a specialized region called a *centromere* ('central thing') that is responsible for the movement of the chromosome into daughter cells. The ends of chromosomes, called *telomeres* ('distant things'), consist of large numbers of short repeat sequences that are maintained independent of replication by the enzyme *telomerase*.

Somatic cells are *diploid*, meaning that each chromosome is present in two copies (one pair). One copy in each pair is derived from the father and the other from the mother. As cells divide, the genome is perpetuated through the process of mitosis. Mitosis is divided into several stages corresponding to events that are visible in the light microscope (see Chapter 1).

> Mitosis copies the genome and distributes all genes to daughter cells. *Meiosis* separates chromosome pairs and distributes single alleles to germ cells.

Fig. 3.1 Meiosis is the process of generating haploid germ cells. One pair of homologous chromosomes is shown. DNA is replicated before meiosis begins. In late prophase, the homologous sister chromatids pair and engage in crossing over, generating recombinants.

Meiosis—forming germ cells

A human germ cell (an egg or a sperm) has 23 *unpaired* chromosomes. Germ cells are thus *haploid*, meaning that only one copy of each chromosome is present. When an egg

MEIOSIS—GERM CELLS HALVE THE GENOME

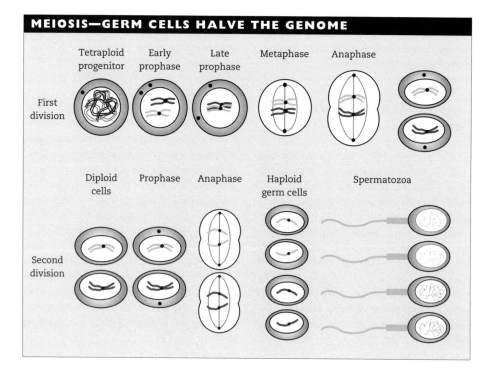

and a sperm unite to form a fertilized ovum or zygote, a new human being with a unique combination of chromosomes is created. In preparation for fertilization, the diploid germ cell progenitors replicate their genomes once and divide twice (meiotic division), which results in half as many chromosomes per (haploid) germ cell.

First meiotic division—copy and divide

Before the first meiotic division, the germ cell progenitors replicate their DNA so that each chromosome is a double structure comprised of two identical *sister chromatids* and the cell contains double the normal amount of DNA (Fig. 3.1). No further DNA replication occurs during meiosis. During prophase, chromosomes condense and become visible, revealing the two identical sister chromatids held together at the centromere. The homologous chromosomes become intimately paired during late prophase. The X–Y chromosomes do not pair except through a relatively small region on the short arms. The exchange of chromatid segments occurs at this stage through the process of *recombination* (Fig. 3.2).

Second meiotic division—divide and consort

After the first meiotic division, each daughter cell contains both sister chromatids of each chromosome. Note that these are not normal diploid cells because the chromatids are identical, except for recombination. During the second meiotic division, the paired chromosome strands divide at the centromere. Each daughter germ cell receives 23 *single* chromosomes, one member of each original chromosome pair (Fig. 3.1).

In males, all four haploid cells develop into sperm. In females, however, only one of the four haploid cells develops into an egg. The other three haploid cells, called polar bodies, are very small cells; this conserves the progenitor cell cytoplasm for a single large egg. The first meiotic division occurs in human females before their birth and the second meiotic division is completed during ovulation, when the

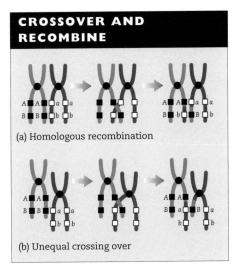

CROSSOVER AND RECOMBINE

(a) Homologous recombination

(b) Unequal crossing over

Fig. 3.2 Recombination occurs where chromatids cross over. (a) Homologous recombination occurs when paired chromatids cross over during prophase in meiosis. Here, two loci are shown with two alleles at each locus (A or a and B or b). Afterward, there are two chromatids of the parental haplotype (AB and ab) and two recombinant haplotypes (Ab and aB). (b) Unequal crossing over occurs when non-homologous regions of the chromosomes pair. The result is two parental chromatids (AB and ab), one chromatid with a gene duplication (Aab) and one with a gene deletion (B).

egg matures. In males, meiosis does not begin until adolescence and continues thereafter throughout adult life.

Genes on different chromosomes have a 50% chance of being inherited together because chromosomes segregate into germ cells independently. Genes on the same chromosome *may* be inherited together, depending on how close they are. The further apart the genes, the greater the chance that they will be separated by recombination (Fig. 3.2). Overall, the chance of recombination is roughly 1% per million base pairs (Mbp). Since chromosomes average 100 Mbp in length, genes on one chromosome often segregate independently. However, recombination does not occur randomly. For example, recombination is particularly common within highly repetitive *Alu* sequences,

ALU IN THE (REPEAT) FAMILY

Alu elements are short (~300 bp), moderately repetitive DNA sequences that are recognized by the restriction enzyme AluI. There are about 300 000 *Alu* sequences dispersed throughout the human genome. *Alu* elements are flanked by direct repeat sequences, thereby resembling transposons, and include a 14-bp sequence that is identical to some viral origins of replication. The function of *Alu* repeats is unknown but they may contribute to genomic DNA replication and promote recombination. For example, recombination between *Alu* repeats in the cholesterol receptor gene causes deletions, resulting in familial hypercholesterolaemia.

raising the possibility that such sequences may be involved in promoting recombination.

> Individuals with identical alleles of a given gene are *homozygous* at that genetic locus. *Heterozygotes* possess two different alleles.

Recombination is the exchange of DNA between chromosomes (Fig. 3.2). Homologous recombination between similar DNA sequences occurs when pairs of condensed chromosomes (chromatids) 'cross over' while they are juxtaposed during prophase. Unequal crossing over results in the deletion of DNA from one chromatid and its duplication on the other. This creates variations in length and may cause the reciprocal loss and duplication of a gene. Multigene families (see p. 68) are thought to have arisen through this process. Breakpoints within genes can also give rise to new genes, formed by the fusion of DNA sequences from both chromosomes. Non-homologous recombination, in which crossing over occurs between different sites on either the same or different chromosomes, is less common. Telomeric repeat sequences protect chromosome ends from recombination.

> Traits encoded by *dominant* alleles are expressed to the exclusion of other alleles. Traits encoded by *recessive* alleles are expressed in homozygotes.

Different genes that are close together on a chromosome and therefore tend to assort together, rather than independently, are said to be *genetically linked*. This forms the basis for performing linkage analysis (see p. 74) to map genes in relation to each other.

Mendelian laws

Mendel summarized his findings in two laws (Fig. 3.3).

1 *Each trait is controlled by two hereditary factors (alleles), which segregate unchanged into different gametes (germ cells).* A heterozygous parent with one dominant and one recessive allele of a given gene, symbolized as *Aa*, generates equal numbers of gametes containing each allele, *A* or *a*. A cross between two heterozygous parents produces 25% *AA* progeny, 50% *Aa* or *aA* progeny, and 25% *aa* progeny.

2 *Hereditary, particulate factors (genes) controlling different traits assort independently.* Parents heterozygous at two different genes (*Aa* and *Bb*) give rise to progeny that have each allele in the same frequency. Only 25% of their progeny would have the same genotype (*AaBb*) as the parents and double homozygotes are the most rare (1/16 = 6%).

These conclusions stood in contrast to the views of Mendel's contemporaries, who believed that parental traits blended in the progeny. Mendel's laws fit our understanding of many gene behaviours.

Patterns of inheritance

Four different patterns of inheritance occur depending on whether the gene is dominant or recessive and whether it is carried on a sex chromosome or an autosome (not X or Y).

1 Autosomal recessive—affects people of either sex whose parents are usually both asympto-

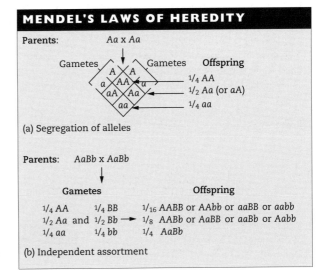

MENDEL'S LAWS OF HEREDITY

Parents: Aa x Aa

Gametes   Gametes   Offspring

A   A
a   AA   a
aA   Aa
aa

1/4 AA
1/2 Aa (or aA)
1/4 aa

(a) Segregation of alleles

Parents: AaBb x AaBb

Gametes   Offspring

1/4 AA   1/4 BB   1/16 AABB or AAbb or aaBB or aabb
1/2 Aa and 1/2 Bb →   1/8 AABb or AABB or aaBb or Aabb
1/4 aa   1/4 bb   1/4 AaBb

(b) Independent assortment

Fig. 3.3 Mendel derived simple laws of heredity.

matic carriers. The risk of having an affected child is increased if the parents are related.

2 Autosomal dominant—affects people of either sex who usually have at least one affected parent.

3 X-linked recessive—almost always affects males whose mother is a carrier. There is no male to male transmission. Females may show some mild disease characteristics because of random inactivation of the X chromosome.

4 X-linked dominant—affects females more often, but usually less severely, than males. There are no known Y-linked diseases.

Fig. 3.4 Pedigree charts demonstrate representative patterns of Mendelian gene inheritance.

Typical Mendelian patterns of inheritance can be demonstrated in families in which a disease can be tracked through several generations (Fig. 3.4).

• Single copies of an *autosomal recessive* allele are carried without effect (phenotype). If both parents are carriers, their children have a 25% chance of being normal, a 25% chance of being affected, and a 50% chance of being carriers. If only one parent is a carrier, the children have a 50% chance of being carriers.

• Even a single copy of an *autosomal dominant* allele influences the phenotype. Children of an affected parent have a 50% chance of being affected.

• The influence of an *X-linked recessive* allele depends on the sex of the individual. In

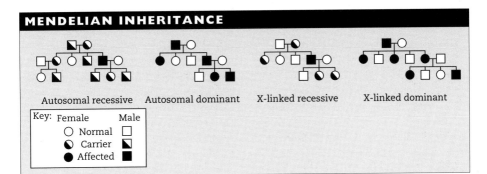

MENDELIAN INHERITANCE

Autosomal recessive   Autosomal dominant   X-linked recessive   X-linked dominant

Key: Female   Male
○ Normal   □
◑ Carrier   ◪
● Affected   ■

X CHROMOSOME INACTIVATION

In females, one of the two X chromosomes is randomly inactivated on day 16 after fertilization, when the embryo consists of 5000 cells. The inactivation of this same X chromosome is maintained in all the progeny of these cells. This results in a mosaic pattern of expression for some genes on the X chromosome. In heterozygous females for example, two different allelic forms of the enzyme glucose-6-phosphate dehydrogenase can be detected in large, contiguous patches of different tissues. (X inactivation in female cats causes similar chimerism that can be readily observed in calico coat colour patterns.) The process of inactivation involves expression of a gene called X-inactivation-specific transcript (*XIST*). *XIST* is expressed exclusively on the inactive chromosome, which condenses and can often be recognized in female cells as a dark staining 'Barr body' on the edge of the nucleus.

females, both X chromosomes must be mutant for a phenotype. In males, the phenotype is manifested when the single X chromosome is mutant. Similarly, daughters of a female carrier have a 50% chance of being carriers while sons have a 50% chance of being affected.
• The inheritance of *X-linked dominant* alleles depends on the sex of the offspring. Sons of an affected male are normal because their X chromosome is from their mother. Daughters of an affected male are always affected because one of their X chromosomes is from their father. Children of an affected female have a 50% chance of being affected.

The differentiated human cell contains 46 chromosomes of which two are sex chromosomes and the remaining 44 are autosomes. The female has two X sex chromosomes, and the male one X and a shorter Y sex chromosome. The autosomes are present in homologous (matched) pairs, so that each one has a partner with the same morphological appearance.

Genomic diversity: how do we differ?

Diversity in the genome arises during the sexual process through the random assortment of chromosomes and through the *crossing over* or *recombination* of DNA between chromosomes. These processes shuffle DNA sequences. Diversity also occurs through novel,

MUTAGENIC CHEMICALS

Several types of chemicals can cause mutations. These include agents that insert (intercalate) into DNA and distort its structure (such as acridine dyes); deaminating agents (such as hydroxylamine); agents that mimic nucleotides and are incorporated, disrupting base pairing; and alkylating agents (such as cyclophosphamide). Exposure to these chemicals increases the chance of mutation.

random changes in the DNA sequence, called *mutations*.

Even though the human genome can be recognized as a distinct set of chromosomes with specific sizes and banding patterns, the DNA sequences and their organization are continually undergoing change, resulting in diversity between individuals. These alterations occur during the sexual process and also arise from errors introduced during DNA replication. DNA mutations can also occur as a result of environmental factors. In 1927, Muller showed that X-rays are powerful agents of mutation (mutagens) in fruit flies. Chemicals can also cause mutation through a variety of mechanisms (see box above).

Genes, loci and alleles

A particular form of a gene is called an *allele* and the position of the gene on a chromosome is its *locus*. Generally, only one or few different alleles exist for any particular gene but some genes are highly polymorphic, meaning that many different alleles exist. When an individual has two identical alleles, they are *homozygous* at that locus. If there is only one allele, such as genes on the X and Y chromosomes, the individual is *hemizygous* at that locus. When an individual has two different alleles, they are *heterozygous* at that locus.

The physical characteristic resulting from expression of a single allele, or the interaction between several alleles, is known as the *phenotype*. A *dominant* allele always contributes to the phenotype. A *recessive* allele needs to be present on both chromosomes (homozygous) to influence the phenotype.

The complexity of genetic organization makes description difficult and the nomenclature is often imprecise. A *gene* is a unit of heredity but the term is actually used synonymously with a length of DNA encoding an RNA and usually a protein. While useful, this simplification ignores the consequence of DNA elements controlling transcription. The more general term *locus* would be perfect if genes always had one order on the chromosome, like points in a line. But DNA moves and mutates, and is duplicated and deleted. Accurate description and understanding is improved by the precise use of these terms.

Genetic variation

Although each chromosome in a pair is morphologically similar, their exact genetic material varies as a result of chromosome recombination and random assortment during meiosis and DNA mutation. The rate of mutation varies throughout the genome. More variation is found in non-coding regions (introns, flanking regions, repetitive DNA sequences), than in protein-coding regions (exons). This may reflect the fact that *surviving* mutations are most likely to occur in 'unimportant' DNA (since most mutations are bad). The highest known mutation rate occurs in repetitive non-coding sequences such as minisatellite regions.

Variations in the DNA sequences of genes *may* alter the protein that is encoded. For example, in sickle cell anaemia (Fig. 3.5) a single base substitution in the β-globin gene (GAG to GTG) leads to glutamic acid being replaced by valine in the β-globin chain of haemoglobin. The resulting haemoglobin molecule (haemoglobin S) differs in structure from normal haemoglobin and promotes sickling of red blood cells. However, alteration of GAG to GAA would still code for glutamic acid, and although the DNA sequence of the gene had changed, the protein product would be the same.

DNA mutations may:
- have no effect on the expression of a gene (be silent);
- change the level of gene expression (increase or decrease);
- produce a related but structurally different protein.

Alternatively, genetic variation may lead to production of different proteins, all of which are regarded as normal. For example, an individual's ABO blood group signifies whether they express A, B or O antigens on their red cells, any combination of which is considered normal.

> Blood group antigens (ABO) are glycolipids and glycoproteins. Their expression depends on the genes encoding the enzymes that synthesize and transfer the carbohydrate chains.

DNA mutations

DNA can be altered (mutated) in various ways.
- *Point mutations* replace one nucleotide with another. Point mutations within coding regions

POINT MUTATIONS

> The most common mutation is substitution of cytosine (C) with thymine (T). This occurs because cytosine, when followed by guanine (CpG), is often methylated to give 5-methyl-cytosine, which is unstable. Deamination of 5-methyl-cytosine yields thymine. Thus, CpG is often replaced by TpG.

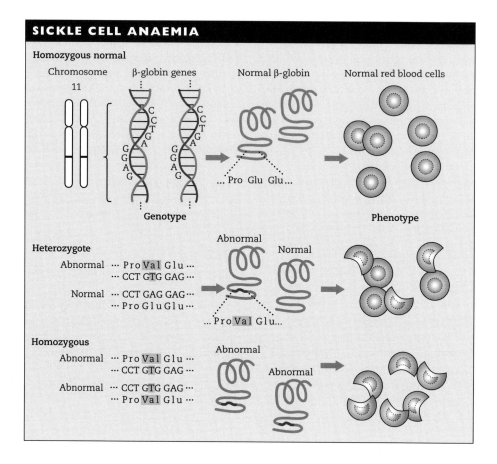

SICKLE CELL ANAEMIA

Homozygous normal

Chromosome 11   β-globin genes   Normal β-globin   Normal red blood cells

... Pro Glu Glu...

Genotype   Phenotype

Heterozygote

Abnormal   ··· Pro Val Glu ···
           ··· CCT GTG GAG ···

Normal   ··· CCT GAG GAG ···
           ··· Pro Glu Glu ···

Abnormal
Normal

...Pro Val Glu...

Homozygous

Abnormal   ··· Pro Val Glu ···
           ··· CCT GTG GAG ···

Abnormal   ··· CCT GTG GAG ···
           ··· Pro Val Glu ···

Abnormal
Abnormal

Fig. 3.5 A point mutation causes sickle cell anaemia. The substitution of a single nucleotide (A → T) in the β-globin gene leads to the replacement of the normal glutamic acid with a valine. The resulting, abnormal haemoglobin protein (haemoglobin S, HbS) differs in structure. When exposed to low oxygen (hypoxia), which is encountered in the peripheral tissues, the red blood cells (RBCs) containing HbS are prone to dramatic shape changes called sickling. These sickled RBCs are less durable and tend to deteriorate, causing anaemia.

may lead to different amino acids being incorporated into the protein or cause premature termination of translation if a stop codon is introduced (Fig. 3.6). Since the genetic code is degenerate (each amino acid is encoded by more than one base triplet), alteration of a single nucleotide may *not* alter the amino acid sequence (be silent). The first and best-known example of a point mutation leading to an altered protein product is in sickle cell disease, which was shown by V. M. Ingram in 1956 (Fig. 3.5). You would expect that such a deleterious mutant would be selected against during evolution, resulting in a low frequency of that allele. However, the abnormal haemoglobin (HbS) that leads to sickle cell anaemia may also protect against some consequences of malaria. This benefit to heterozygotes may protect the allele encoding HbS.

• *Deletions or insertions* alter both the length and sequence of DNA. Reciprocal mutations in chromosome pairs may result from unequal crossing over during meiosis. Deletions from single chromosomes can occur when a loop

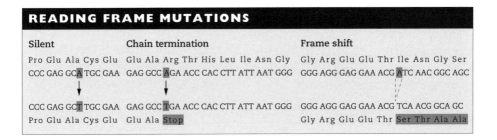

READING FRAME MUTATIONS

Silent	Chain termination	Frame shift
Pro Glu Ala Cys Glu	Glu Ala Arg Thr His Leu Ile Asn Gly	Gly Arg Glu Glu Thr Ile Asn Gly Ser
CCC GAG GCA TGC GAA	GAG GCC AGA ACC CAC CTT ATT AAT GGG	GGG AGG GAG GAA ACG ATC AAC GGC AGC
↓	↓	
CCC GAG GCT TGC GAA	GAG GCC TGA ACC CAC CTT ATT AAT GGG	GGG AGG GAG GAA ACG TCA ACG GCA GC
Pro Glu Ala Cys Glu	Glu Ala Stop	Gly Arg Glu Glu Thr Ser Thr Ala Ala

Fig. 3.6 Small mutations within a protein-coding sequence can dramatically alter the protein. Mutations in the third nucleotide in a codon are often silent, meaning that the protein is not changed. Mutations producing a premature stop codon lead to truncated proteins. Frameshift mutants usually completely change the subsequent amino acids.

forms during DNA replication, which is lost when the two ends reunite (Fig. 3.7a). Deletions and insertions range from a single base to several megabases. Large deletions can result in the loss of whole genes. Small deletions or insertions in the protein-coding portion of a gene usually change the reading frame, resulting in *frameshift mutations* and proteins with truncations or dramatically changed sequences (Fig. 3.6). Ionizing radiation and mutagenic chemicals increase the spontaneous chromosomal breakage rate. Deleted fragments that lack a centromere are lost during subsequent cell division.

• *Inversions* reverse the order of genes in a chromosome. This occurs when the chromosome is broken at two places and the intervening segment is reinserted back-to-front (Fig. 3.7b). As with translocation, DNA is not usually lost but genes may be disrupted at the breakpoints or brought under control of different regulatory sequences.

• *Translocations* reposition large chromosomal fragments within the genome. Recombination between non-homologous chromosomes or breakage of two chromosomes followed by abnormal repair results in the rearrangement of large portions of the genome (Fig. 3.7c). There is usually no loss of DNA. However, bringing a gene under the control of different regulatory sequences can dramatically alter its expression.

The consequence of a mutation depends on whether it occurs in egg or sperm (germ) cells or in differentiated tissues.

• Germ cell mutations do not lead to abnormalities in the affected individual, but can be inherited and cause disease in subsequent generations.

• Somatic cell mutations in differentiated tissues are not inherited, but may lead to disease

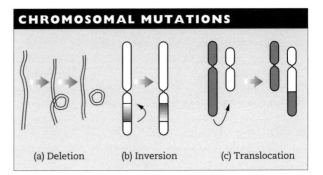

Fig. 3.7 Chromosome scale mutations can be detected by karyotyping. Large changes can be detected by missing or rearranged chromosome bands. A deletion from chromosome 11 causes Wilms' tumour. A translocation from chromosome 8 to 14 causes Burkitt's lymphoma.

CHROMOSOMAL MUTATIONS

(a) Deletion   (b) Inversion   (c) Translocation

MANY DIFFERENT MUTATIONS CAUSE THALASSAEMIA

Alpha thalassaemia is usually caused by large deletions in the α-globin gene, although a minority of cases are caused by more subtle mutations. Beta thalassaemia is caused by various different point mutations or small deletions in the control regions, reducing transcription, or splice sites, altering mRNA processing, resulting in abnormal, reduced or absent β-globin production. Major deletions in the β-globin genes are rare.

in the affected individual. Such mutations are of particular importance in the development of cancer.

Some diseases are always caused by a mutation in one particular gene (monogenic). Sickle cell anaemia results when a point mutation alters a single amino acid in the β-globin chain of haemoglobin. However, many different mutations in the α- or β-globin genes give rise to thalassaemias.

Evolution of the human genome

Although evolution leads to the accumulation of many differences, the human genome contains DNA sequences that are closely related to those of other species. These DNA sequences appear to have been 'conserved' during the process of evolution. For example, genes encoding histone proteins are remarkably similar in different species.

Gene families

Genes with similar structure and function (gene families) occur throughout the human genome. Genes that are similar are said to be *homologous*. Strictly speaking, homology is more than similarity because it suggests an evolutionary link between two or more genes or proteins. Homologous proteins that perform the same function in different species are called *orthologues*, while those that perform different but related functions in one species are called *paralogues*.

Gene families may be clustered together, such as the five β-like globin genes on chromosome 11 (Fig. 3.8) or dispersed throughout the genome (ribosomal RNA (rRNA) genes are found on five different chromosomes). Some families stay close, others drift apart. Histone

β-GLOBIN GENE FAMILY

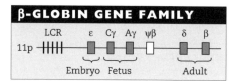

Fig. 3.8 The genes of the β-globin family are clustered on the short arm of chromosome 11. The different β-globin genes are ordered in the sequence in which they are expressed during development. ε-Globin is made very early in embryonic development, the two γ-globin variants are expressed during fetal life, and the δ- and β-globin genes take over after birth. A pseudogene is indicated by ψ. The locus control region (LCR) is a group of (tissue-specific) enhancers that activate transcription in erythroid cells.

genes are clustered at a few locations on chromosomes 1, 6 and 12. Gene families often contain pseudogenes (ψ), which are similar in structure to functional members of the gene family but are themselves inactive because of alterations in their regulatory sequences, coding regions, or both.

The existence of gene families suggests that the human genome has evolved from successive alterations, rearrangements and duplications of DNA.

Repeated sequences and 'junk'

The human genome has an immense coding capacity: enough to encode more than a million different proteins the size of haemoglobin. However, the existence of large families of repeated sequences within the genome was suggested by early studies that analysed the rate at which melted DNA reanneals. Recent evidence from the human genome sequencing project suggests that perhaps only 30 000 genes are encoded within the genome. Some of the extra DNA seems to have no function, so-called 'junk' DNA. The remainder is re-peated sequences that may or may not have function. Different families of repeats have been identified based on their:

• number—total number of repeats in the genome;
• motif—presence of core repeat sequences;
• distribution—dispersed or grouped together in the genome;
• structure—presence of flanking ('terminal') repeats and their orientation (direct or inverted);
• length—ranging from single nucleotides to kilobases; and
• location—association with particular sites, such as centromeres, telomeres or hete-rochromatin.

One such family is the *Alu* family of repeats that were introduced above. *Alu* repeats are short, they display a distinct sequence motif, they are moderately repetitive, they are dis-persed throughout the genome with no clear associations, and they are flanked by direct repeats.

Moderately repetitive DNA comprises approximately 30% of the genome. Some repeated sequences have clear functions. For example, ribosomal RNAs are repeated up to 2000 times (5S subunit) and transfer RNAs are repeated approximately 1300 times.

Satellite DNA

Highly repetitive DNA comprises approxim-ately 25% of the genome. Some highly repetit-ive sequences have no known function. They form large arrays that were originally called *satellites* because they form a distinct peak upon caesium chloride density separation due to their content of G-C nucleotides. Subsets of satellites can be classified according to their sequence motifs, length and size (Table 3.1).

Satellite DNA is typically not transcribed and forms the bulk of heterochromatin (chro-matin that remains condensed during inter-phase). The *hypervariable* family of minisatellite DNA shares a sequence motif and is dispersed. The number of these repeats at any given locus varies, thereby forming one method of

Table 3.1 Characteristics of repetitive, satellite DNA.

SATELLITE DNA			
Repeat name	**Repeat size**	**Total size**	**Features**
1 Satellite	5–200 bp	Up to several million bp	Found in heterochromatin and centromeres Not transcribed
2 Minisatellite (a) Hypervariable family	10–60 bp	1000–20 000 bp	Share a common core sequence (motif) GGGCAGGANG (where N is any base), dispersed, VNTRs
(b) Telomeric family	6 bp	1000–20 000 bp	Usually TTAGGG and repeated about a thousand times Protects chromosome ends
3 Microsatellite	1–4 bp	Less than 1000 bp	Repeats of A and CA are the most common Dispersed throughout genome

bp, base pairs; VNTRs, variable numbers of tandem repeats.

identification called *variable numbers of tandem repeats* (VNTRs). The *telomeric* family of minisatellite DNA almost certainly protects the chromosome ends from random recombination events. Microsatellite DNA consists of runs of dinucleotide repeats, most commonly CA (or TG on the complementary strand), that are dispersed throughout the genome.

Variations in the number of minisatellite repeats between individuals can be detected by using a restriction enzyme that cuts outside an array of repeats. These variations give rise to different-sized DNA fragments, which can be separated in a gel and detected by hybridization with a probe that recognizes the repetitive unit. With the exception of identical twins, there are variations in minisatellite regions between all individuals, and these variable regions are inherited in a Mendelian fashion. This forms the basis for the technique of DNA fingerprinting, in which the size of minisatellite regions at numerous loci is determined by probing restriction fragments of total DNA.

Trinucleotide repeats

A novel form of genetic mutation involves the amplification of a DNA sequence that contains repeats of three nucleotides (trinucleotide repeats). The repetitive sequences are also present in the genes of normal individuals but they are amplified up to a thousand-fold in the genes of affected patients. Diseases which result from the amplification of trinucleotide repeats include:

• myotonic dystrophy—a progressive muscle weakness in which there is continued muscle contraction of muscles after cessation of voluntary effort;
• fragile X syndrome—X-linked intellectual disablement (mental retardation);
• Huntington's chorea—progressive dementia and involuntary movements in middle age;
• X-linked spinobulbar muscular atrophy (Kennedy's disease)—muscle weakness associated with testicular atrophy and gynaecomastia;
• spinocerebellar ataxia type 1.

Trinucleotide repeat sequences occur in both protein-coding and untranslated regions

of genes. The myotonic protein kinase gene normally has between five and 40 repeats of the trinucleotide CTG in its 3′ untranslated region. In patients with myotonic dystrophy, up to 3000 CTG repeats have been found in the same region of the gene. In Kennedy's disease (X-linked spinobulbar muscular atrophy), there is amplification of a CAG repeat in the first exon of the androgen receptor gene.

The total length of the trinucleotide repeat sequence tends to increase as the gene passes from parent to offspring, providing a molecular explanation for *anticipation*, the phenomenon by which a disease gets progressively more severe through successive generations.

DNA fingerprinting

Although there is variability between genes of different individuals, most variation occurs in the non-coding regions of DNA. These regions, rather than genes themselves, can be used to create unique genetic 'fingerprints' that help to navigate around genetic maps. For example, polymerase chain reaction (PCR) amplification of VNTRs located 'upstream' (5′) of the human insulin gene on chromosome 11 (11p15.5) can be used to distinguish alleles that are positively associated with type I diabetes, alleles that are dominantly protective, and a third allele that is rare.

Identifying genetic differences

Restriction fragment length polymorphism (RFLP)

This powerful method of identifying genetic differences is classical, i.e. it is understood by the old-timers. DNA treated with a restriction endonuclease is cut at specific sequences or *restriction sites* (see Chapter 2). In the case of genomic DNA, this produces a large number of *restriction fragments* of many different lengths. Any changes in the sequence within the restriction site, which would block cutting, or changes in the distance between restriction sites, such as the number of repetitive sequences, changes the restriction fragment length. Thus, RFLP is a sensitive measure of genetic

RFLP—RESTRICTION FRAGMENT LENGTH POLYMORPHISM

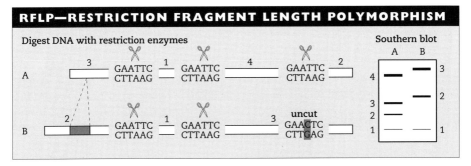

Fig. 3.9 Genetic variations can be identified by restriction fragment length polymorphism (RFLP). DNA is digested with a restriction endonuclease (here, *Eco*RI), then Southern blotted. The DNAs labelled A and B differ in two ways: A has three restriction sites while B has two, and an insertion (or deletion) has occurred within one fragment. These differences are reflected in the pattern of bands on the Southern blot. Although several bands are shown on the Southern blot, typically only a single gene would be detected with a labelled probe.

variation between two individuals (Fig. 3.9). RFLPs were used to map the gene on chromosome 7 that when mutant causes cystic fibrosis.

Polymerase chain reaction (PCR) in genetic analysis

Once a region that is suspected of carrying a mutation has been identified, further analysis usually depends on the use of PCR to amplify large quantities of the DNA segment from normal and affected individuals.

Several methods can then be used to determine whether an individual carries a mutation.

• The primers can be designed so that one overlies the mutation. If the primer matches the normal DNA sequence, amplification will occur in normal individuals, whereas if the primer matches the mutated sequence, amplification occurs in affected individuals. For example, the amplification refractory mutation system (ARMS) distinguishes mutant and normal alleles (see Fig. 3.15, p. 80). Amplification would occur with both primers with template DNA from a heterozygous individual.

• The DNA segment can be amplified using primers that match sequences outside the region of mutation, and the DNA product ('amplicon') analysed for the mutation using a separate procedure. For example, products of normal and mutant genes can be distinguished by single-strand conformation polymorphism (SSCP) (see Fig. 3.16, p. 81).

For example, the PCR products can be hybridized to labelled oligonucleotide probes that recognize either the normal or mutated sequence. Alternatively, if the mutation creates or destroys a restriction site, the amplified product can be examined to determine whether it is cleaved by the restriction enzyme.

Randomly amplified polymorphic DNA (RAPD)

Randomly amplified polymorphic DNA (RAPD) markers are created by the PCR amplification of random sites in the genome (Fig. 3.10). A single oligonucleotide, usually 10 nucleotides long, is used to prime the amplification of genomic DNA. The primer need not anneal perfectly. At a relatively low annealing temperature the oligonucleotide will anneal at many locations in the genome. However, because only one primer is used, amplification products will be generated only when complementary (inverted) repeat sequences occur in close proximity (generally less than 2000 bp). Each primer will generate a different pattern and mixing primers can increase the complexity of the pattern. Although easy to perform, amplification can be very sensitive to the exact reaction conditions, with different patterns

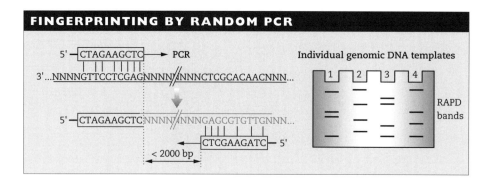

FINGERPRINTING BY RANDOM PCR

Fig. 3.10 Fingerprinting by degenerate PCR. Annealing of a short primer of arbitrary sequence to random complementary sites in the generation of random amplified polymorphic DNA (RAPD). Some of the bands amplified by a random primer are polymorphic, revealing differences between individuals.

generated depending on the annealing temperatures and even the model of thermocycler. A number of similar techniques go by other names, such as arbitrarily primed PCR (AP-PCR).

The number and size of the amplification products will vary in different regions of the genome, and will vary between individuals. With some randomly chosen primers no sequences will be amplified. With others some PCR products of the same length, and others of different length, may be generated from DNA of different individuals. Bands that vary in size are randomly amplified polymorphic DNA (RAPD) bands. This identification method is most reproducible when applied to relatively simple genomes such as those of the pathogens *Trypanosoma cruzi*, which causes trypanosomiasis, and *Staphylococcus aureus* (staph A).

Amplified fragment length polymorphism

Amplified fragment length polymorphisms are detected using a combination of restriction digestion and PCR amplification. Genomic DNA is first cut with both a restriction enzyme that cuts frequently (*Mse*I which has a 4-bp

recognition sequence), and one that cuts less frequently (*Eco*RI, which has a 6-bp recognition sequence). Adaptor molecules which recognize the cut ends are then joined onto the fragments, allowing amplification of subsets of restriction fragments using primers specific for different adaptor molecules. The process is more complicated than other methods, but yields more mappable polymorphic loci for each reaction.

Finding genes: maps, markers and mutants

As more disease-causing mutations are identified, accurate diagnosis may increasingly depend on the detection of gene mutations. Even simple genome variations, where no direct consequences are known, may be useful for locating genes and finding contributing genes. These uses have prompted the development of improved techniques for mutation and variation detection.

Here, we will first review the basic methods used to analyse genes. Some of these tools may be of only historical interest as the map of the human genome is essentially complete. A review will help to understand how the forest was assembled from the trees.

Genome maps—getting physical

Genetic maps were under construction long before it was known *what* should be mapped physically. The first mapping determined only

MAPS: GENETIC AND PHYSICAL

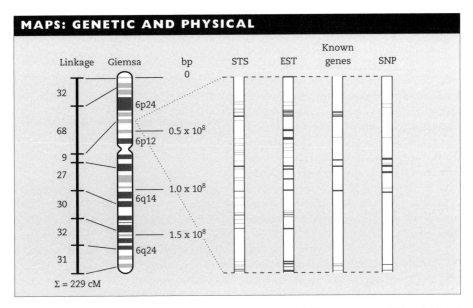

Fig. 3.11 Mapping genes onto chromosomes. Here are several maps of chromosome 6, which contains 189 279 554 bp. Linkage maps measure distance by the frequency of recombination (cM). Early physical maps measured distance in banding patterns on Giemsa-stained chromosomes. Current maps measure distance in nucleotides. An expanded view of the 6p21.33 band is centred on nucleotide 33 500 000 (0.335 × 10^8), approximately the position of the human histocompatibility gene HLA-A. Within this band, sequence tagged sites (STS), expressed sequence tags (ESTs, only those with introns) and single nucleotide polymorphisms (SNPs, only those from overlaps) are listed. Data are from the Cooperative Human Linkage Center and draft human genome sequence (October 2000), which was interpreted with the genome browser at University of California, Santa Clara (genome.ucsc.edu).

whether genes are close to each other, also known as *linked*. Two genes are said to be linked when they are usually inherited together. Closer genes are less likely to be separated by recombination, which therefore becomes a measure of distance. A recombination rate of 1% (1 crossover in 100) is called a centimorgan (cM), named by J. B. S. Haldane for T. H. Morgan, who started mapping fruit fly genes in the early 20th century. It was soon apparent that genes are arranged linearly, even those in a circle, such as mitochondrial or bacterial genes.

One centimorgan (1 cM) represents on average about 1 million base pairs (1 Mbp) of DNA. However, sites of recombination are not random, and thus the actual physical distance represented by a centimorgan varies

according to whether recombination occurs more or less commonly in the region of interest (compare the linkage map to the physical map in Fig. 3.11).

Genetic linkage maps

The earliest genetic maps were linkage maps. The closer together that the markers for two different characteristics lie on the same chromosome, the less likely that a recombination event will occur between them, and separate them, during meiosis. Markers that are close together will tend to be tightly linked, and passed together from parent to child.

Inherited characteristics that differ between individuals (allelic differences) occur in coding sequences (exons) and in non-coding sequences, which include regions within genes (introns) and regions between genes that regulate their expression. Some differences can be detected by their influence on physical characteristics, such as eye colour. However, most differences occur in non-coding sequences that are detected by molecular techniques, such as analysis of repeated regions (microsatellite), sequence-tagged sites (STSs), or single nucleotide polymorphisms (SNPs). Collaborative efforts of over 100 laboratories resulted in the publication (1994) of the first high-resolution, comprehensive human linkage map. It consisted of 5840 loci (mostly microsatellite regions) with an average distance of 0.7 cM between them.

LINKAGE–LOD VALUES

The probability of a genetic linkage is calculated by statistical analysis, usually by computer, and is expressed as a lod (logarithm of the odds) score. Lod values of less than 3 (representing a probability of 1000/1, as lod scores are base 10) are generally taken as evidence of linkage.

Transcriptome–cDNA (transcript) maps

The most interesting part of the genome has long been thought to be the genes that encode mRNAs, which are translated into proteins. A comprehensive effort to sequence all mRNAs, in the form of complementary DNAs (cDNAs), was started in the early 1990s. All of the cDNA clones obtained from a particular tissue represent a library of the genes that were expressed when the tissue was obtained. In 1994, an international consortium was formed to construct a physical human gene map of cDNA-based, *expressed* sequence-tags (EST). By 1998 a map of 30 181 human gene-based markers had been assembled and integrated with genetic maps produced by radiation hybrid mapping (see box opposite). This map includes most genes that encode proteins of known function.

Mapping directions—forward and reverse genetics

If the DNA sequence of the gene is known, then the gene can be physically mapped to a specific chromosomal region by a process known as *forward genetics*. In the recent past, this would involve cloning larger regions of chromosomal DNA, which would be sequenced and positioned by looking for STSs. It is now possible to simply compare the cloned sequence to the entire sequence of the human genome. Query sequences can be submitted over the internet to powerful computer programs (e.g. BLAST, basic local alignment search tool) that quickly search the genome databases (e.g. GenBank or EMBL) and return matches.

If the only information about a gene is the physical characteristic (phenotype) it produces, then the gene can be mapped by a process known as *reverse genetics*. This approach is based on the odds of two genes being inherited together; the chances are greatest if they are close together on the same chromosome, whereas recombination through successive generations is more likely to separate genes that are further apart. Cloning a gene when nothing is known about it except its location is known as *positional cloning*.

A series of tests (known as *linkage analysis*) is performed to test the association of the phenotype with known markers. The association is tested in pedigrees, testing the likelihood that the genes are inherited together. These markers are usually known genes or physical markers such as RFLPs, STSs or ESTs. The strength of linkage (probability) is measured by LOD (*logarithm of the odds* score; see box above).

The region of interest can then be examined for evidence of functional genes. Once a candidate gene has been identified, it is cloned and sequenced. The amino acid sequence of the protein product can be deduced and the cloned gene can be expressed in an artificial expression system.

Somatic cell hybridization

One method for localizing genes to particular chromosomes is *somatic cell hybridization*. This

technique exploits the fact that when human
and rat cells are fused, the resulting hybrid cells
randomly lose chromosomes, producing cells
in which only some human chromosomes are
present. These cells can then be screened for
the presence of either a known DNA sequence (using a labelled cloned DNA fragment),
or the protein product of a specific gene.
Alternatively, the donor cell can be irradiated,
which causes chromosomal breakage (radiation hybrid; see box above).

Sequence-tagged sites (STSs)—unique tags in the genome

Reference points that can be easily identified
are needed at numerous sites when con-
structing maps of the genome. Such landmarks
are provided by sequence-tagged sites (STSs).

STSs are sequences in the genome that can be
uniquely amplified by PCR. They serve as
markers in genetic mapping, allowing smaller
pieces of DNA to be aligned and combined
into larger physical maps. Conditions for PCR,
including the primer sequences, buffers and
temperatures, are available on the internet.
For example, over 3000 STSs are defined for
the approximately 180 000 kb of chromosome
6, an average of one STS per 60 kb (see also
SNPs, p. 80).

If an STS is part of a coding DNA region, it is
known as an expressed sequence tag (EST).
ESTs are usually obtained by sequencing a fragment of a cDNA clone.

Molecular gymnastics—chromosome walking and jumping

A particular region of chromosome can be
explored by walking or jumping (Fig. 3.12).

In *chromosome walking* (Fig. 3.12) a DNA
fragment that contains the starting point (the
marker that has been linked to a gene) is
isolated from an appropriate library that contains overlapping regions of genomic DNA.
The fragment is then used to find other cloned
fragments that overlap with it. By repeating
this procedure it is possible to 'walk' in steps

Fig. 3.12 Chromosome
neighbourhoods can be
characterized in detail by
walking or crudely by jumping.
Both approaches identify a
flanking clone in a library using
a probe from a known region
(Probe 1). Walking probes can
be made by sequencing to the
unknown end of the fragment
(crawling) or by using
restriction enzyme fragments
after the sites are mapped.
Jumping probes are made by
circularizing the fragment,
which juxtaposes the two ends.
By priming from the known
end, the unknown end (Probe 2)
can be sequenced, skipping the
intervening fragment DNA.

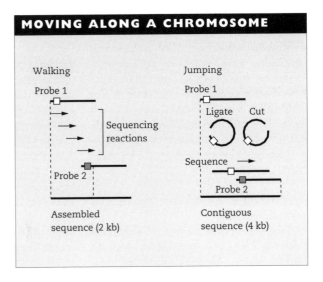

MOVING ALONG A CHROMOSOME

Walking

Probe 1

Sequencing
reactions

Probe 2

Assembled
sequence (2 kb)

Jumping

Probe 1

Ligate   Cut

Sequence

Probe 2

Contiguous
sequence (4 kb)

HTF–GENE SCREEN

HpaII tiny fragments (HTF) islands, also called CpG islands, are short stretches of DNA which are often found at the 5′ end of genes. HTF islands are rich in unmethylated CpG dinucleotides and can be readily identified because they are cut into tiny fragments by the restriction enzyme HpaII, which recognizes the sequence CCGG.

created by each new fragment along the chromosome.

Chromosome walking involves characterizing every fragment from the starting point to potential candidate genes. Large intervening sequences can be skipped by *chromosome jumping* (Fig. 3.12) in which large fragments of DNA with a marker at one end are sized and then circularized so that the two ends are brought together. The circle is then itself cut into fragments, one of which now contains the marker linked to a sequence a measured distance away.

Potential genes can be identified within large stretches of DNA by looking for *Hpa*II tiny fragments (*HTF*) *islands* (see box above). The restriction enzyme *Hpa*II ('hoppa 2') cuts in the sequence CCGG only when both cytosines are unmethylated. CpG dinucleotides in the mammalian genome are typically methylated, probably as either a consequence or cause of transcription inactivity, but CpG dinucleotides near active genes are often unmethylated. Therefore, *Hpa*II cuts genomic DNA much more frequently near active genes. Note that methylation patterns are *lost* when DNA is cloned (see *Restriction and modification*, p. 36), so the screen must be performed directly on genomic DNA prepared from mammalian cells.

Artificial chromosomes—bacterial (BACs) and yeast (YACs)

Plasmids are excellent for cloning kilobases of DNA (see Chapter 2). Cosmids are very large plasmids that can be used for cloning larger fragments (up to 45 kb). Cosmids also contain *cos* sites (cohesive sequences), which allows them to be packaged into bacteriophage particles for more efficient subcloning and identification. Fosmids are similar to cosmids but potentially more stable because they are maintained as only a single copy per cell.

A *library* is a collection of clones, usually mixed together, that each represent small parts of a more complex whole.

Limitations on the size of DNA fragments that can be cloned into vectors have been overcome by incorporating large fragments of human DNA into *yeast artificial chromosomes* (*YACs*). Complete genomic DNA libraries can be created by fractionating human chromosomes, inserting fragments of up to 2 million bp in length into YACs, and growing them in yeast (*Saccharomyces cerevisiae*). More recently the development of bacterial artificial chromosomes (BACs) has facilitated completion of the Human Genome Project. BACs are propagated as stable inserts in bacteria (*Escherichia coli*), and are usually about 150 kbp in length. A database of the sequences of the ends of BAC clones has been created, providing a framework to link DNA sequences over large regions. These DNA libraries can then be used to create physical maps of *contig*uous sequences (contigs) of human chromosomes.

Finding genes

The location of genes can be determined by using the techniques of genetic mapping (linking genes to other genes), and physical mapping in which the exact chromosomal location is defined. The exact approach depends on how much is known about the gene of interest.

The simplest approach is to sequence the region of interest, but this is slow and only able to analyse several hundred nucleotides from a known sequence in the genome. Large-scale mapping relies on a simple notion: genes that are physically close are more likely to stay together.

DNA SEQUENCING

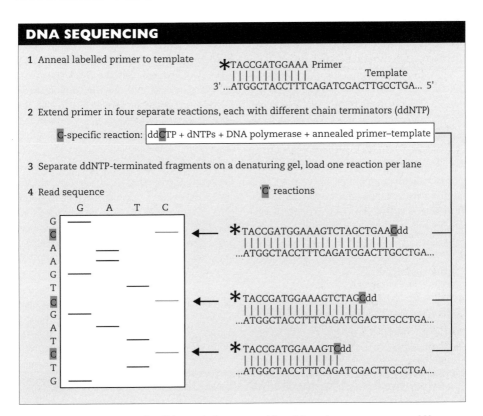

1 Anneal labelled primer to template

✱TACCGATGGAAA Primer
|||||||||||||
3' ...ATGGCTACCTTTCAGATCGACTTGCCTGA... 5' Template

2 Extend primer in four separate reactions, each with different chain terminators (ddNTP)

C-specific reaction: | ddCTP + dNTPs + DNA polymerase + annealed primer–template |

3 Separate ddNTP-terminated fragments on a denaturing gel, load one reaction per lane

4 Read sequence   'C' reactions

G A T C

G
C
A
A
G
T
C
G
A
T
C
T
G

✱TACCGATGGAAAGTCTAGCTGAACdd
|||||||||||||||||||||||||||||
...ATGGCTACCTTTCAGATCGACTTGCCTGA...

✱TACCGATGGAAAGTCTAGCdd
|||||||||||||||||||||
...ATGGCTACCTTTCAGATCGACTTGCCTGA...

✱TACCGATGGAAAGTCdd
|||||||||||||||
...ATGGCTACCTTTCAGATCGACTTGCCTGA...

Fig. 3.13 DNA sequencing using dideoxy chain terminators is also known as Sanger sequencing. Note that only a fraction of each reaction is terminated by the addition of dideoxynucleotide (ddNTP) at each corresponding nucleotide position. Otherwise, no sequence would be obtained beyond the first nucleotide. Fluorescent nucleotides are often used instead of a radioactive primer.

DNA sequencing

> DNA is sequenced to determine the order of the nucleotides.

There are two ways to sequence DNA, the hard way using noxious chemicals or the modern way using enzymes and inexpensive kits. (Then there is the easiest way, using a commercial service.) These methods involve four nucleotide-specific reactions that remain incomplete, each reaction yielding a heterogeneous population of molecules that terminate at one particular nucleotide. The enzymatic method of sequencing, also called

Sanger sequencing after its developer, uses dideoxynucleotides (ddNTPs). Unlike normal deoxynucleotides (dNTPs), dideoxynucleotides cannot be extended by DNA polymerase. These populations of molecules are then resolved on a denaturing polyacrylamide gel, one lane per nucleotide-specific reaction (Fig. 3.13).

A modification of the DNA sequencing technique uses a thermostable polymerase, as used in PCR, and repeatedly anneals, extends and melts. Although no chain reaction is established in this procedure because the product does not act as template in the next round, it can provide a sequence from very little DNA template. The elevated extension temperature also reduces interference from secondary structures in the template and simplifies sequencing double-stranded DNA.

In chemical sequencing, also called *Maxam–Gilbert* sequencing after the developers, the sequence is obtained from the DNA itself, instead of an enzymatic copy. The DNA to be sequenced is labelled at one end and then treated with chemicals that specifically destroy one or two of the nucleotides (either purines or pyrimidines or only one nucleotide). The reactions are not allowed to go to completion, otherwise only the shortest product would remain and no sequence 'ladder' would be obtained.

Southern blotting

A Southern blot is performed to identify and to determine the size of a DNA fragment.

Southern analysis involves separating DNA fragments on a gel, blotting the gel and then hybridizing the blot with a labelled probe (Fig. 3.14). The gel separates the DNA fragments according to size and the hybridization step provides specificity in detection, allowing the identification of DNA fragments. For example, to determine the size of the genomic *Eco*RI fragment(s) containing the β-globin gene, one would cut genomic DNA with *Eco*RI, separate the resulting fragments on an agarose gel, blot and probe with a fragment of the β-globin gene. Alternatively, to test whether a PCR-amplified product is what you think it is, you might blot it and probe the blot with a labelled fragment of the gene.

An important application of Southern blotting is in pedigree analysis (Fig. 3.14b). Testing whether offspring are carriers of genes that predispose to or cause disease, and paternity testing are two examples of this analysis.

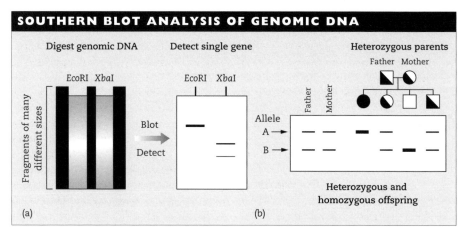

SOUTHERN BLOT ANALYSIS OF GENOMIC DNA

(a)   (b)

Fig. 3.14 Southern blots analyse DNA sequences. (a) Genomic DNA is digested with restriction enzymes. On the left is the EtBr-stained agarose gel showing the heterogeneously sized fragments of digested genomic DNA (the average length is a function of the recognition site size). After blotting, the gene is detected on one *Eco*RI fragment and two smaller *Xba*I fragments, meaning that the gene is flanked by *Eco*RI sites and there is an *Xba*I site within the gene. (b) Southern blots can help in pedigree analysis. In this example, digestion of genomic DNA with a restriction enzyme produces different-sized fragments. This is known as restriction fragment length polymorphism (RFLP). If the larger fragment (indicated with black in the pedigree) were associated with a disease, such an analysis would strongly suggest close monitoring of the first offspring (the daughter represented by a filled circle). The second and fourth offspring are carriers of the disease-associated gene and the third offspring does not carry the disease-associated allele (the son represented by an open square).

Genomic DNA is cut with a restriction enzyme and blotted and the blot is hybridized. Either the restriction enzyme or the probe distinguishes between the alleles of the gene.

Pulsed field gel electrophoresis —the old standard

Initially, the techniques for mapping genes were limited by the size of DNA fragments that could be separated by gel electrophoresis. Regular gel electrophoresis (see Chapter 2) cannot separate large pieces of DNA. Pulsed field gel electrophoresis (PFGE) overcomes this problem. Periodically changing the direction of the electric field ensures that DNA will not snake through the gel. When genomic DNA is cut with restriction enzymes with 8-bp recognition sequences, very large sequences of DNA are produced.

Fluorescent in situ hybridization —go FISH

Fluorescent in situ hybridization (FISH) localizes genes on chromosomes with light. Probe oligonucleotides, DNA or RNA, are labelled with fluorescence and then annealed to a spread of metaphase chromosomes. FISH decoration of metaphase (condensed) chromosomes give nice pictures that look like bright-eyed worms. FISHing with probes from known locations in the genome, such as STSs (see p. 75), on interphase chromosomes can resolve genes that are separated by as little as 50 kb. Whole chromosomes can be 'painted' different colours with probes that anneal to chromosome-specific sequences.

FISH can be used in diagnosis. Amplification of the HER-2/neu gene on chromosome 17 is associated with poor prognosis in breast cancer. FISH with a HER-2/neu probe can distinguish amplified and normal genes.

Comparative genomic hybridization (CGH), a variation on FISH, can be used for whole genome analysis. Normal genomic DNA is labelled with one colour fluor and test genomic DNA is labelled with a second fluor. These DNAs are both hybridized to an array of probes (see also Gene chips, p. 86). Excess normal genomic DNA competes with the test genomic DNA so that only genomic regions that are amplified in the test genome produce detectable hybridization.

Finding mutants

The importance of finding mutants or variants will increase as more diseases are linked to specific genes or mixtures of genes. A number of diseases caused by monogenic mutants have been identified. Predisposition to complex diseases such as hypertension can also be linked to certain mutations.

The most straightforward way to find variants is to sequence the DNA, of course. This has been such a slow, tedious method that an eminent scientist once proposed sentencing criminals to sequencing kilobases of DNA instead of years in prison. However, new machines with very high capacity ('throughput') may change these considerations, making the following just a historical overview.

Single nucleotide resolution by PCR

Amplification refractory mutation system (ARMS)
Single nucleotide differences can be resolved in PCR (Fig. 3.15). This method relies on the differential speed with which Taq DNA polymerase extends a matched versus a mismatched primer. An oligonucleotide primer with even a single nucleotide mismatch at the 3′ end is extended by DNA polymerase only very inefficiently. Normal and mutant alleles may be easily distinguished. The situation shown in Fig. 3.15, where the normal allele acts as template and yields a product, could be easily reversed. With a primer matching the lower template, product would rapidly accumulate with this template.

Single nucleotide primer extension (SNuPE, 'snoop', minisequencing) is a variant of ARMS. SNuPE uses four different primers, each with a different nucleotide at the 3′ end at the SNP. The primers that match the SNPs are extended, and this can be measured ('scored') in different ways. This method can also be applied to the microarray format.

SINGLE NUCLEOTIDE RESOLUTION BY PCR

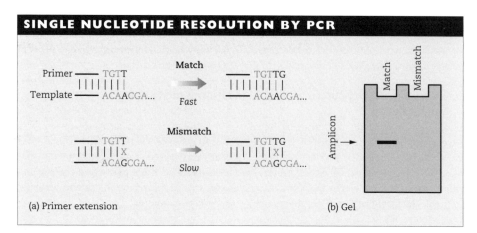

(a) Primer extension   (b) Gel

Fig. 3.15 Single nucleotide variants can be distinguished by DNA polymerase in the amplification refractory mutation system (ARMS). (a) DNA polymerase rapidly extends a primer that perfectly matches the template (above) while a mismatched primer is extended only slowly (below). (b) Repeated primer extensions in PCR amount to large differences in product accumulation.

Single-strand conformation polymorphism—mutants in the amplicon

Single-strand conformation polymorphism (SSCP) is a quick way of finding mutants in relatively big pieces of DNA (Fig. 3.16). Single-stranded DNA tends to fold into a complex structure, which in part determines the mobility of the DNA strand in a non-denaturing gel. PCR is used to amplify the fragments that contain the suspected polymorphism, then the fragments are labelled, denatured by heating, and then rapidly cooled to encourage annealing between regions of the single strands. Strands snap back and form regions of intrastrand annealing, which migrate differently through a gel. Even a single base change in the DNA can alter this conformation, and hence the mobility of the DNA sequences on a gel.

Single nucleotide polymorphism (SNP, 'snip')

Single nucleotide polymorphism (SNP) is a conceptual tool that focuses attention on even the smallest differences in gene sequences (polymorphisms). Often, approaches to detecting polymorphisms identify only particular subsets of sites or relatively large changes. For example, only changes that occur within a restriction endonuclease recognition site can be detected by RFLP analysis. SNPs ignore the techniques by which differences are detected and together constitute the personal genome sequence.

> Variations in a single base pair occur on average once every 1000 bp throughout human DNA. These differences are known as single nucleotide polymorphisms (SNPs).

SNPs can be used as markers to identify susceptibility genes that regulate individual responses to disease or drugs. Rare or unique SNPs might be useful for identifying individuals, but the SNPs most useful for mapping studies occur in approximately 1% of individuals. This frequency allows rapid mapping because many individuals possess the SNP. In tests, SNPs have proven capable of locating genes involved in several diseases, including sickle cell anaemia, psoriasis, migraine, Alzheimer's and diabetes.

The SNP Consortium was formed to create and make available a high quality map of the variations that occur in individual base pairs throughout the human genome. The SNP consortium is a non-profit organization whose

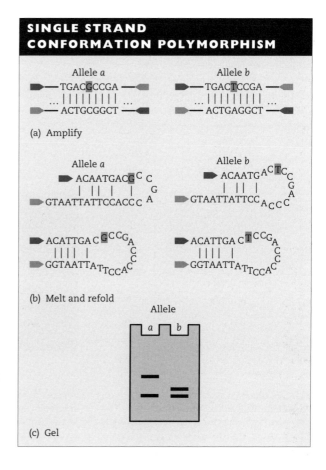

Fig. 3.16 Single-strand conformation polymorphism (SSCP) can find variants in amplicons. After amplification (a), labelled PCR products are melted and rapidly cooled (b), encouraging single-stranded folding through intrachain annealing. The single nucleotide difference between the alleles causes some folded forms to have loops of different sizes (upper forms) while others are unaffected by the mutation (lower forms). (c) A gel resolves the different folded forms.

members include a number of pharmaceutical and computer companies, as well as the Sanger Centre and the Wellcome Trust in the UK and in America the Whitehead Institute and the Washington University School of Medicine. The SNP Consortium will collaborate with the Human Genome Project to identify SNPs. This collaborative effort will sequence DNA from 24 anonymous donors with diverse geographical origins, providing a rich source for SNPs. As SNPs are identified they will be validated, mapped and made available through a publicly accessible database, called dbSNP.

Gene expression: RNA analysis

A gene is said to be *expressed* when the product is made and is functional, which requires gene transcription and transcript processing. Mutations in the genetic regions that control these processes can profoundly alter the expression of a gene.

Northern blot

Northern blots are used to identify, quantify, and determine the size of a mRNA species.

In a Northern analysis, RNA molecules of different sizes are resolved on a denaturing formaldehyde-containing agarose gel, the gel is blotted and the blot is hybridized with a labelled probe (Fig. 3.17). The denaturing gel unfolds the RNA so that separation is based on length alone and not on secondary structure such as hairpin loops. The formaldehyde in the

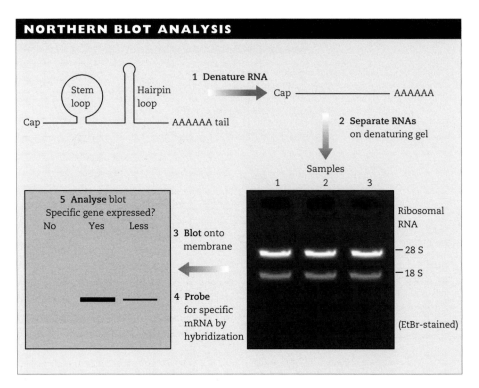

Fig. 3.17 Northern blots analyse gene expression. RNA is typically denatured by treatment with formamide then size separated on a denaturing agarose/formaldehyde gel. Along with quantifying the amount of mRNA, mRNA size can be estimated by comparison to the ribosomal RNA (rRNA) or to size standards run in a separate well. Using less stringent probe hybridization conditions could also test the expression of similar genes (homologues).

gel reacts with the denatured nucleotides and prevents their refolding. The formaldehyde is soaked out of the gel and away from the RNA before blotting.

Nuclease protection assay

Nuclease protection assays are used to measure mRNA and analyse mRNA structure.

Certain nucleases can digest only single-stranded nucleic acids; double-stranded nucleotides are not digested. This forms the basis of the nuclease protection assay where mRNA, which is single stranded, is hybridized to a single-stranded probe. The hybridized part of the probe is resistant to treatment with single-strand-specific nucleases (Fig. 3.18). There are two major types of nuclease protection, depending upon whether the probe is RNA or DNA:

• *RNase protection* assay—the unhybridized part of an *RNA probe* is digested with RNase A and RNase TI; and

• *SI nuclease protection* assay—the unhybridized part of a *DNA probe* is digested with SI nuclease.

Although the nuclease protection assay entails more work than a Northern blot, it has certain advantages for analysis of mRNA levels, including the following:

• mRNA fine *structure can be analysed* because the probes can distinguish even single nucleotide differences;

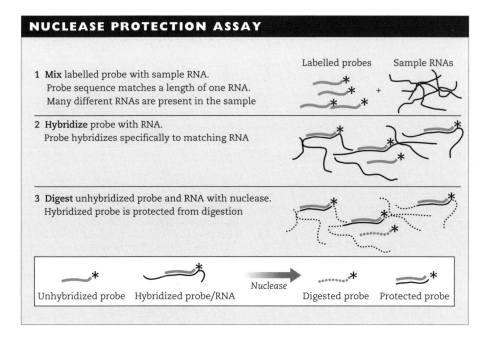

NUCLEASE PROTECTION ASSAY

Labelled probes   Sample RNAs

1 **Mix** labelled probe with sample RNA.
Probe sequence matches a length of one RNA.
Many different RNAs are present in the sample

2 **Hybridize** probe with RNA.
Probe hybridizes specifically to matching RNA

3 **Digest** unhybridized probe and RNA with nuclease.
Hybridized probe is protected from digestion

Unhybridized probe   Hybridized probe/RNA   *Nuclease*   Digested probe   Protected probe

Fig. 3.18 The nuclease protection assay provides a sensitive quantification of mRNA. Excess probe is added and hybridized to the RNA (steps 1 and 2). The amount of the probe protected from digestion by nuclease depends on the amount of matching RNA (step 3). Intron/exon junctions and transcription start sites could also be mapped with probes that overlap the junctions.

• it is *more quantitative*, because solution hybridization is well defined in physiochemical terms (kinetics, temperature of hybridization) but blotting is not;
• *less RNA* can be used (2–5 μg total RNA versus 5–20 μg for a Northern);
• somewhat *degraded RNA can be analysed* because only a small portion of the RNA is hybridized.

Complementary DNA (cDNA) cloning

A clone is a population of genetically identical organisms, cells or molecules that derive from the replication of a single progenitor. cDNA is the reverse complement of mRNA, which encodes proteins. All mRNAs possess a poly(A) tail (a string of A ribonucleotides that is added to the 3′ end of mRNA after transcription), whereas ribosomal RNA (rRNA) or transfer RNA (tRNA), which make up the bulk of total or cytoplasmic RNA preparations, do not. Oligo dT (a string of T *deoxyribonucleotides*) is often used to prime the first strand synthesis by RT, because it anneals specifically to the poly(A) tail and can thereby selectively prime cDNA synthesis from mRNA (Fig. 3.19). The second strand is more difficult to synthesize and several methods have been developed.

DNA cloning is the production of multiple identical copies of a DNA fragment.

Here are several reasons why cDNA cloning is popular and powerful.
• cDNA is shorter than the gene. Some relatively small proteins are encoded by incredibly large genes, possessing long introns and untranslated regions (UTRs). Dihydrofolate reductase (DHFR), for example, has a protein-coding

cDNA CLONING

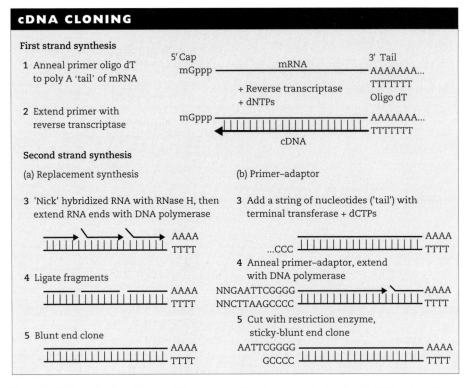

First strand synthesis

1 Anneal primer oligo dT to poly A 'tail' of mRNA

2 Extend primer with reverse transcriptase

Second strand synthesis

(a) Replacement synthesis

3 'Nick' hybridized RNA with RNase H, then extend RNA ends with DNA polymerase

4 Ligate fragments

5 Blunt end clone

(b) Primer–adaptor

3 Add a string of nucleotides ('tail') with terminal transferase + dCTPs

4 Anneal primer–adaptor, extend with DNA polymerase

5 Cut with restriction enzyme, sticky-blunt end clone

Fig. 3.19 cDNA can be cloned by two different methods. Synthesis of the first cDNA strand is primed by oligo dT, which anneals to the poly(A) tail of mRNA. Second strand synthesis is more difficult and two of the many different protocols are shown. (a) Replacement synthesis is simple but the extreme 5′ end is lost because there is no primer further upstream to replace the RNA. Ligation proceeds despite this RNA end and the cap. (b) The primer–adaptor method is more complicated but it can clone the 5′ end. For this method, the oligo dT primer in the first strand synthesis often also contains a restriction site, which permits directional cloning into expression vectors.

region of approximately 600 bp distributed over a gene that is 31 500 bp.

• cDNA contains all the important parts. The exons are usually the more interesting part, at least initially, because their sequence affords what is often the first glimpse into what the protein looks like.

• cDNA can be made from RNA that is enriched for the mRNA of interest by using particularly high expressing cells or by treating cells to induce the mRNA, whereas for the genomic sequence only two copies are present in each and every (somatic) cell.

Recombinant proteins

Recombinant DNA technology allows the production of large quantities of pure proteins for clinical practice and research. The proteins produced by these techniques are termed recombinant even when they are identical to the natural proteins. Many recombinant human proteins are used in clinical practice (see Chapter 4).

Once the gene for a particular protein has been cloned, it is inserted into plasmid under the regulation of a strong promoter. Such a construct is called an *expression vector* because it is designed to express large amounts of protein. Different promoter sequences are used depending upon whether the protein is to be made in bacterial, yeast or mammalian cells. The expression vector encoding the recombinant protein is then transfected into the genome of microorganisms or cultured mammalian cells, which then produce the protein.

Making mutants

Mutants are invaluable for determining the function of a gene or protein. Entire signalling pathways can be probed in whole cells using random mutagenesis. Precise mutations of genes can probe the function of individual regions. Individual amino acids can be changed with site-directed mutagenesis, yielding proteins that are more useful.

Fig. 3.20 Site-directed mutagenesis can be used to redesign a protein. Here, the recognition site for the complement enzyme factor Xa, is mutated. The resulting protein is not cleaved and might be more stable *in vivo*.

Site-directed mutagenesis—designer genes

> Site-directed mutagenesis is used to prepare specific mutants (variants) of a known gene.

At last, here is an art, in the form of biotechnology, that improves on nature. Natural mutants are generated *randomly*, through mistakes in DNA synthesis or repair, and most are deleterious. The rare beneficial mutation could still be lost unless it happens to be very beneficial, such as when the alternative is extinction. Even with accelerated mutagenesis and screening/selection *in vitro*, this is too slow, far too slow, for your biotechnologist 'on the go'. Synthetic oligonucleotides are the answer for quick (and, with PCR, easy) designer genes (Fig. 3.20).

Microbial pharmacists

Recombinant proteins are finding more uses in medicine and more are promising. An intriguing approach avoids the pharmaceutical paradigm by instead altering normal bacteria to

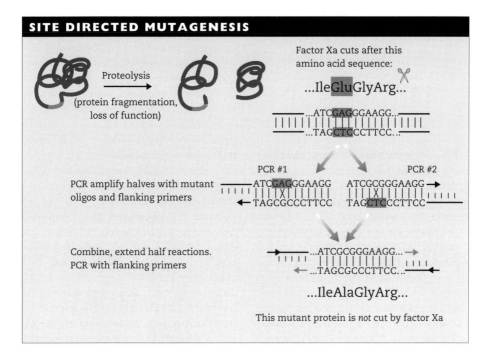

SITE DIRECTED MUTAGENESIS

Proteolysis
(protein fragmentation, loss of function)

Factor Xa cuts after this amino acid sequence:
...IleGluGlyArg...

...ATCGAGGGAAGG...
||||||||||||||||||||
...TAGCTCCCTTCC...

PCR #1   PCR #2

PCR amplify halves with mutant oligos and flanking primers

ATCGAGGGAAGG
||||||X||||||
TAGCGCCCTTCC

ATCGCGGGAAGG
||||X||||||
TAGCTCCCTTCC

Combine, extend half reactions. PCR with flanking primers

...ATCGCGGGAAGG...
||||||||||||||||
...TAGCGCCCTTCC...

...IleAlaGlyArg...

This mutant protein is *not* cut by factor Xa

produce beneficial proteins *in situ*. One report claims to have cured inflammatory bowel disease (in mice) by administration of non-pathogenic, non-invasive and non-colonizing bacteria (*Lactococcus lactus*) that were engineered to secrete the immunomodulatory protein interleukin 10 (IL-10).

Reverse transcriptase–PCR (RT–PCR) assay

> Reverse transcriptase–PCR (RT–PCR) is used to detect very small amounts of mRNA.

Retroviruses use reverse transcriptase (RT) to convert their RNA genomes into DNA. When coupled with PCR amplification, RT can provide the only means of measuring very small amounts of RNA, much less than is necessary for a northern blot or even a nuclease protection assay. The RNA is reverse transcribed by RT using oligo dT or six-base oligonucleotides with random sequence ('random oligos') that anneal all over the RNA. These act as primers that are extended to produce a cDNA strand, which is then amplified by PCR.

> 1 Make cDNA from RNA with RT and oligo dT primers.
> 2 PCR amplify cDNA with gene-specific primers.
> 3 Analyse PCR products.

RT–PCR is excellent for determining whether a gene is transcribed and it can be used to measure large differences in mRNA levels, but it is poor at reliably measuring smaller differences (10-fold and less). This is because slight differences in the efficiency of PCR amplification produce large differences in product, independent of the original amount of template. For example, the difference between an efficiency of 80 and 85% yields a difference of more than six-fold after 30 cycles ($1.6^{30} = 1.3 \times 10^6$ versus $1.7^{30} = 8.2 \times 10^6$). A modification, called *competitive PCR*, controls for differences

in amplification efficiency by including in every sample different, known amounts of a distinguishable template (Fig. 3.21). The point in the titration at which the cDNA and the added competitor template produce an equal amplification is then taken as a measure of the original cDNA amount.

Note that the absolute amounts of the competitor and cDNA are not necessarily the same at the equivalence point, but they are amplified to yield equivalent amounts of product. Different efficiencies of amplification may occur when the sequences are different (one is preferentially amplified). One sequence may be shorter or contain lower G/C content, which is copied more easily because of the lower bond strength. Competitive PCR has the advantage of allowing comparisons to be made in the *plateau phase* of the amplification, where sufficient product has accumulated to allow easy detection. The products of regular PCR can be compared only in the *exponential phase* of amplification, which is tedious to determine, and the products are difficult to detect. The lesser template quickly 'catches up' in the plateau phase and reduces any original differences.

Gene chips—parallel analysis

Large-scale measurement of the genome provide the 'big picture' that can permit distinctions to be made even when it was not known (a priori) what exactly was different. This strategy, in other words, is to look everywhere and figure out what you're looking for later. A trend toward miniaturization, which allows small sample volume and high sample 'throughput', where analyses are performed quickly, suggests that gene chips are the analytical tools of the future (Fig. 3.22).

Instead of probing many different genes in one sample, it is also possible to probe many different samples with one gene. Gene chips may be made with immobilized copies of a patient's genes, which are then probed with oncogenes or other disease-related genes. For example, chips have been used to detect mutations in the cystic fibrosis gene (*CFTR*), a breast cancer gene (*BRCA1*) and the oncogene p53.

QUANTITATIVE PCR

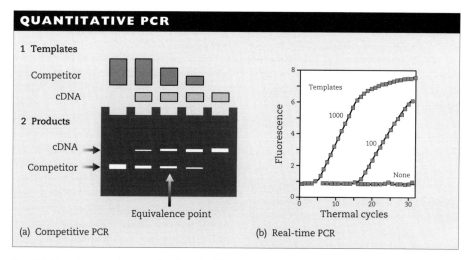

(a) Competitive PCR

(b) Real-time PCR

Fig. 3.21 Templates can be quantified by PCR. (a) In competitive PCR, a constant amount of cDNA and a known amount of competitor template is added to each reaction. Control reactions at each end contain only competitor template or cDNA. The products are analysed on an agarose gel. The equivalence point, where the intensities of the competitor and cDNA bands are equal, is a measure of the specific RNA from which the cDNA was generated. (b) Real-time PCR is performed in special thermocyclers that can read fluorescence. With more templates in the initial mixture, the product accumulation is detectable earlier.

GENE MICROARRAYS—ANALYSIS IN THE CHIPS

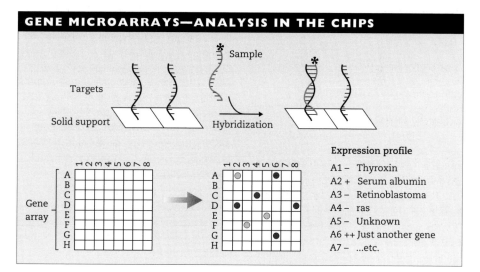

Fig. 3.22 Gene 'chips' can identify transcripts. The sample nucleic acid (DNA or RNA) is often marked with a fluorescent dye. The target DNA is bound to solid support, forming 'features'. The array of genes would actually be very large, often thousands of different genes. RNA and synthetic oligonucleotides can also be used as sample or target material. The genes arrayed on the chip may be chosen for particular profiles, such as a tumour characterized for the expression of tumour suppressors and oncogenes.

The classification of cancers such as melanoma has benefited from the ability to assess the global gene expression simultaneously throughout the genome.

Serial analysis of gene expression (SAGE)—one tag at a time

As attractive as 'gene chips' are, the future of gene expression studies may actually use a technology that is less immediately tractable. Serial analysis of gene expression (SAGE) relies on the fact that a short (10–24) nucleotide sequence can uniquely identify any given transcript (mRNA). These sequences act as a 'tag'.

These tags can be linked together, cloned, sequenced and analysed efficiently by machine. By counting the incidences of any particular tag, the frequency of the corresponding transcript can be measured.

Gene modulation and modification

RNA interference (RNAi)—kill the messenger

Double-stranded RNA can *silence* homologous genes through RNA interference (RNAi).

Genes can be silenced post-transcriptionally through a phenomenon, called RNA interference (RNAi), that is still somewhat mysterious. When a double-stranded RNA (dsRNA) molecule is injected into a cell, mRNAs that are homologous (roughly 80%) to the injected dsRNA are degraded by nucleases. An RNA-dependent RNA polymerase is involved, perhaps in generating the templates that direct digestion of the homologous RNAs. The natural, physiological function of RNAi might be to suppress endogenous retrotransposons, which depend on transcription for their mobility, and foreign genes such as viruses. This phenomenon is being actively developed to probe gene function by mani-pulating gene activity.

Antisense oligonucleotides—block translation or destabilize message?

Antisense suppresses gene expression by blocking translation of the mRNA or by destabilizing the mRNA.

Antisense suppression is where the expression of a protein is inhibited by the annealing of a matching (complementary) RNA or synthetic oligo to a sequence within the mRNA, thereby blocking or reducing the efficiency of translation (Fig. 3.23). Getting antisense RNA into the cell usually means first transfecting the gene in the reverse orientation (so that it is read 3′–5′), and then getting it expressed at high levels, both of which are difficult tasks. Since this method uses a large part of the gene in reverse orientation, it is also called antigene suppression.

Antisense oligonucleotides are much easier than antigenes to produce and test. Their small size and the ability to attain high concentrations (micromolar) extracellularly may be important for getting effective doses into the cell. However, experimental controls for what is often a very large amount of antisense oligo must include the sense oligo and non-sense oligo (the same nucleotides in a random order). Along with physically blocking translation, the annealed oligo may also function to reduce protein expression by rendering the mRNA susceptible to degradation by RNase H, which is specific for RNA/DNA hybrids (a heteroduplex).

Newer approaches (yet)

Peptide nucleic acids (PNAs)—less repulsive oligos

Peptide nucleic acids (PNAs) are oligonucleotides that are joined together by peptide-like amide bonds instead of the phosphodiester bonds found in natural nucleic acids.

ANTISENSE OLIGONUCLEOTIDES CAN SUPPRESS PROTEIN EXPRESSION

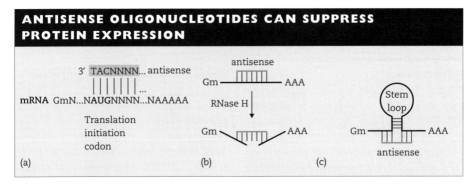

Fig. 3.23 Antisense oligonucleotides (oligos) may reduce protein expression by blocking translation or destabilizing the mRNA. (a) An antisense oligo annealed to the translation initiation site can physically block the movement of the ribosome along the mRNA during translation. An oligo annealing elsewhere to the mRNA may also be effective in suppressing gene expression, either by blocking translation of the full-length protein or (b) by targeting the mRNA for digestion by the RNA/DNA hybrid-specific nuclease, RNase H, or (c) by stabilizing a secondary structure.

ANTISENSE TECHNOLOGY

Although antisense technology has shown promise in blocking the expression of some genes in tissue culture, many oligos that should bind to a particular mRNA fail to block expression of the protein. These failures may be due to the folding of RNA into secondary structures, such as hairpin loops, that exclude the oligo. Alternatively, oligo-induced stabilization of such secondary structures may be necessary to inhibit translation. The imprecision of RNA secondary structure predictions and the inability to control the stringency of mRNA/DNA oligo annealing inside the cell (37°C and physiological salt conditions) may continue to limit the application of oligo-based antisense suppression techniques.

The binding of PNA to DNA is stronger than is DNA to DNA because there are no phosphates on the PNA to repel the phosphate backbone of the DNA and weaken the hybridization. Accordingly, the PNA–DNA or PNA–RNA binding is much less dependent upon the salt concentration of the solution, because there is no charge repulsion that requires shielding with higher ionic strength. PNAs are also relatively resistant to both nucleases and proteases. The term PNA is actually a misnomer because the phosphate backbone (the acidic portion of DNA) is not found in the PNA. The increased strength of hybridization and stability may lead to a role for PNA in antisense inhibition of gene expression.

Aptimers—nucleic acids shape up

Aptimers are nucleic acids that fold into structures that specifically bind other molecules, such as proteins, through interactions that are based on the conformation (shape) of the aptimer rather than a particular sequence of nucleotides. Such interactions may occur naturally in certain complexes between RNAs and proteins (ribonucleoproteins).

DNA sequences have also been designed to bind particular proteins. This approach was discovered by accident when the mechanism of antisense oligonucleotide inhibition was investigated. Surprisingly, the oligonucleotide was found to bind directly to the agonist (a protein hormone) rather than block gene expression. Aptimers may have therapeutic applications in replacing antibodies that can be strongly immunostimulatory (antigens).

Triplex-forming oligonucleotides —gene repair

Oligonucleotides with long runs of purines or pyrimidines, such as GAGAGA binding with TCTCTC, have been shown to form triple-stranded structures. These are stabilized by hydrogen bonds involved in conventional 'Watson–Crick' base pairing as well as the less familiar Hoogsteen base pairing of a second pyrimidine strand. Such triplexes might have a role in gene expression and recombination.

Triplex-forming oligonucleotides (TFOs) have been designed that anneal to specific sequences in the genome and modify gene function. Specific gene mutations in somatic cells have been increased five-fold by treatment of mice with TFOs. In addition, a transcription control region in the γ-globin gene has been efficiently mutated in TFO-treated normal human fibroblasts. Mutation of this silencer increased γ-globin gene expression in erythroid cells, demonstrating a novel approach to treating sickle cell disease by maintaining fetal haemoglobin expression.

Group II introns—targeted transposons

Group II introns are 1.8-kb RNAs that insert directly into genomic DNA and are then reverse transcribed into DNA. These functions are performed by a single intron-encoded protein that has multiple enzymatic activities, including reverse transcriptase, RNA splicing and DNA endonuclease. Insertion of the ribonucleoprotein follows pairing between the intron RNA and a 14-nucleotide sequence within the target DNA as well as interactions between the protein and DNA. This mobile genetic element is found naturally in yeast mitochondria and some bacteria.

The well studied group II intron of the bacterium *Lactococcus lactis* has been adapted to specifically target genes in cultured human cells; the gene encoding the HIV-1 coreceptor (*CCR5*) and an HIV-1 gene encoding polymerase. It remains to be seen whether geno-

mic DNA can be efficiently targeted by group II introns.

Genomics: big picture genetics

The Human Genome Project— thinking big

The Human Genome Project (HGP) was established to determine the complete sequence of the nuclear genome (sequencing of the mitochondrial genome was completed in 1994). At its inception, the HGP was coordinated by the National Institutes of Health (NIH) and US Department of Energy, which has a long history of sponsoring genetic research into DNA damage from radiation and chemicals. The Human Genome Organization (HUGO) was founded in 1989 to promote international collaboration between the scientists involved in the HGP.

On 26 June 2000 the HGP public consortium announced that it had assembled a 'working draft' of the DNA sequence of the human genome, representing the vast majority of our genetic blueprint. The draft, since updated, is freely available on the internet. The approximately 3.1 thousand million (3.1×10^9) bp genome sequence, nearly 90% of which was sequenced by the international HGP, is composed of hundreds of thousands of fragments of varying lengths. On the same day, a private company named Celera Genomics announced its own first assembly of the human genome sequence, which was made fully available only to subscribers. These working drafts are invaluable aids to identifying all human genes and understanding how they are organized and regulated.

The public HGP consortium and private Celera project took different approaches to sequencing and assembling the human genome. If the sequence were printed in this type, it would be over 10 000 km long. Analysing such large genomes involves cutting the DNA into fragments that are small enough to be sequenced. Determining *where* a sequence occurs in the genome then becomes as important as the sequence itself. In the HGP, large fragments of DNA of *known* position were sheared into small fragments, which were then sequenced and reassembled on the basis of sequence overlaps. Sequencing of different regions was coordinated between laboratories to avoid duplicating work. Celera used a 'whole-genome shotgun' strategy in which the genome is randomly broken up into small fragments that are cloned (facilitated by BACs), sequenced, and then put back together again in the correct order. This process was enabled by new, extremely high capacity sequencing machines and sophisticated computer analysis that identified and aligned overlapping sequences.

The creation of maps with reference points throughout the whole genome is an important, intermediate goal of the genome sequencing effort. These genome maps take two forms:
• Genetic maps describe the position of genes or other identifiable DNA sequences, such as restriction length polymorphisms (RFLPs) and microsatellite markers.
• Physical maps rely on variations in the chemical characteristics of DNA. The banding pattern of Giemsa-stained chromosomes (G-bands), which can be observed by light microscopy, represent a low-resolution physical map.

In addition to funding sequencing work, a portion of the estimated $3 billion budget has been committed to the study of the ethical, legal and social implications of genome research, the creation of research training posts, and the development of informatics capable of handling the accumulated data.

Eight major goals were set for the period 1998–2003:
1 completing the human DNA sequence;
2 improving sequencing technology;
3 studying human genome sequence variation;
4 developing technology for functional genomics;
5 completing the sequence of *Drosophila* and starting the mouse genome;
6 encouraging the consideration of ethical, legal and social implications;

7 expanding studies in bioinformatics and computation; and
8 training genome scientists.

What's next?—editing and annotation

The working drafts reported in June 2000 cover 97% of the human genome with an average accuracy of 97%. The next stage is to 'finish' the sequence by filling in the gaps and increasing the overall accuracy to 99.99% (1 error in 10 000). This has already been achieved for chromosomes 21 and 22.

The 'finished' sequence of 33.5 million bp that make up the DNA of chromosome 22 was reported in December 1999. The sequence has an error rate of less than 1 in 50 000 bp and contains only 11 gaps, which cannot be filled using current technology. The location and size of each gap has been identified. At least 545 genes and 134 pseudogenes (genes that no longer function) were identified, and an additional 200–300 genes are predicted. The genes range in size from 1000 to 583 000 bp, with a mean size of 190 000 bp. A large portion of the chromosome (39%) encodes the exons and introns, which are copied into RNA, but only 3% encodes protein. Several gene families that are distributed over large chromosomal regions appear to have arisen by tandem duplication. Regions where recombination was increased, and others where it was suppressed, were also identified. The finished sequence of chromosome 21 was announced in May 2000.

The identification of important sequences within the genome is termed annotation. This difficult process is crucial to making the sequence useful, much in the way that roads are improved by placing signposts and directions. Many known genes are already located in the genome and the sequences of these genes, which are usually of very high quality, were often used to improve the genome sequence. A complete sequence of a human genome is valuable for understanding the genetic basis of evolution, development and disease. However, even a perfect genome sequence will not represent a catalogue of genes.

The genome sequence is *not* a catalogue of genes.

The term 'gene' was coined by W. Johannsen (1909) for each of the units of heredity that control the expression of a trait. The best known examples of genes are DNA sequences that encode single polypeptides. However, genes can also encode molecules that are *not translated* and perform their function as RNAs. For example, ribosomal RNAs are essential elements of cells that are encoded by multiple copies of the genes. Enzymatic RNAs called *ribozymes* have also been characterized in several organisms. Moreover, transposed DNA that is *not transcribed* can modify the expression of a protein, thereby acting as a gene (heritable trait). Even a single gene might have many traits, depending on what is apparent, and several genes can also encode a single trait.

Genes are hard to find in even a relatively short DNA sequence. The rules for identifying the start and end of a gene from the sequence are not known. The interrupted nature of genes complicates identification further. The gene for factor VIII, for example, is encoded within a 200-kb region of DNA by 26 exons comprising less than 3% of the contiguous genomic sequence. The RNA-encoding portion of the genome will be determined by comparison to the EST sequences derived from RNA libraries.

The human genome diversity project

The 'working draft' of the human genome is a major step towards understanding what makes us human. It will also help us to understand what makes each human an individual. The HGP is sequencing DNA obtained from a small number of individuals in North America and Europe who are predominantly of European ancestry. The selection of these individuals should be of little consequence, as it has been estimated that 99.9% of the human genome is identical between individuals. This uniformity makes us all human. It is minor variations in

sequence that help make us all different, can predispose some to disease, and underlie genetic variability in response to treatment.

The human genome diversity project aims to collect DNA from diverse populations across the world and make it available for genetic studies. This process should facilitate the understanding of human diversity, both normal variation and that responsible for inherited disease. However, the project has been criticized on the grounds that it might violate the rights of indigenous people.

Identifying diversity in our genome may also help to define our origins. For example, analysis of variations in mitochondrial DNA has shown greater diversity in Africans than other populations. The world's population appears to have begun with a small group in Africa that migrated around the world. Genetic differences also suggest that the adoption of farming in Europe coincided with the immigration of peoples from the Middle East.

Comparative genomics

The genomes of many different organisms have been sequenced (Table 3.2). They range in size by a factor of one million. The number of genes contained within the larger genomes is only an informed guess because of the difficulty in clearly identifying a gene. However, several families of genes can be clearly identified in many different organisms. For example, several well described signalling pathways are conserved in flies and vertebrates, including transforming growth factor β (TGF-β) and several receptor tyrosine kinase pathways. Many components of these pathways are also found in the worm *Caenorhabditis elegans*.

The complete genomes of more than 13 pathogens have been published and many more are in progress. These sequences will be invaluable tools in the rational development of new vaccines and the evaluation of old vaccines. For example, the complete genome of *Mycobacterium tuberculosis*, the cause of tuberculosis, was published in 1998. Comparison of the genes expressed by different strains of *M. bovis*, which is used in live, attenuated forms as

Table 3.2 A wide range of genomes encode a diversity of life.

COMPARATIVE GENOMICS

Organism	Form	Genome (Mbp)	Cells	Genes
1 pUC19	Synthetic	0.003	(1)	2
2 SV40	Primate virus	0.005	(1)	5
3 M13	Bacteriophage	0.007	(1)	10
4 λ	Bacteriophage	0.05	(1)	66
5 Mycobacterium pneumoniae	Mycobacterium	0.82	(1)	677
6 Mycobacterium tuberculosis	Mycobacterium	4.4	(1)	3918
7 Escherichia coli	Bacterium	5	1	4289
8 Saccharomyces cerevisiae	Yeast	12	1	6200
9 Caenorhabditis elegans	Worm	97*	1000	18 400
10 Drosophila melanogaster	Fruit fly	180*	10 000	13 600
11 Homo sapiens	Mammal	3100*	~200 000 000 000	30 000–150 000?

* Haploid values are shown (most somatic cells have twice as much DNA). Genome size is given in millions of base pairs (Mbp).
(1) pUC19 is a synthetic cloning plasmid. (2) Simian virus 40 (SV40) is a papovavirus that infects monkeys. (3,4) Bacteriophages M13 and lambda (λ) are viruses that infect bacteria. (5,6) Mycoplasm is an intracellular microbe. M. pneumoniae is one cause of pneumonia. (6) M. tuberculosis causes tuberculosis. (7) E. coli is a common laboratory and intestinal bacterium. (8) S. cerevisiae is baker's yeast. (9) The nematode C. elegans was the first multicellular organism whose genome was sequenced. (10) The fruit fly D. melanogaster continues to provide important insights into gene function. (11) Mouse and human genomes are about the same size.

a vaccine against M. tuberculosis, has identified sets of genes that are necessary for effective vaccination and provided an important criterion for evaluating vaccine production. The cholera genome was sequenced with the goal of understanding the biology of the pathogen and creating more effective vaccines.

Model organisms
The pace of the HGP has been accelerated by parallel studies on a number of model organisms, through both the sequence information and the advances in technology they have provided.

The study of the yeast, worm and fly has been justified to taxpayers and donors by claiming that these organisms would tell us a lot about our own biology. The genome sequencing projects have supported this expectation. Out of 289 genes linked to diseases in humans,

177 are also found in the fruit fly, where it has proven much easier to establish the precise function of genes. There also appears to be a core set of genes for eukaryotes. Yeast, which is the simplest single-cell eukaryote, shares 3000 genes with worms and flies. Completion of the human genome will allow even more powerful comparisons of normal and pathological gene function.

Flies and mice with genetically caused lesions in dopamine neurones even display some traits of Parkinson's disease, supporting the hope that these simpler animals can be studied to gain insight into complex human diseases. Transgenic mice that overexpress human α-synuclein, a protein implicated in Parkinson's disease, develop cytoplasmic inclusions that resemble those seen in the human disease.

Completing the sequence of the human genome represents only one step, albeit a large one, towards understanding how cells and organisms work. The enormous task of identifying genes and control regions within the sequence and determining their function is the next challenge. These functions will be aided by comparisons with simpler organisms that perform some of the same tasks.

Haemophilus influenzae—first free-living organism

The bacterium *Haemophilus influenzae* was the first free-living organism for which the complete genome was sequenced (1995). The approach involved the sequencing and assembly of unselected pieces of DNA ('shotgun') from the whole genome. Total DNA was sheared into fragments that were cloned in plasmids using *Escherichia coli* that were deficient in recombination and restriction functions. This created a library of *H. influenzae* DNAs. Approximately half of the plasmid DNA templates were sequenced from both ends while the remainder was sequenced for shorter lengths. Overlapping sequences, identified by computer analysis, were then used to assemble the sequence of the entire genome. A variety of techniques were employed to close gaps before the final sequence was edited by visual inspection. The genome is estimated to contain approximately 1700 genes.

Saccharomyces cerevisiae—first eukaryote

The complete sequence of the yeast *Saccharomyces cerevisiae* was reported in 1996 under the title 'life with 6000 genes'. This was the first full sequence of a eukaryotic genome and is usefully compared to the human genome. Yeast provides an excellent, simple cell model for understanding the functions of genes involved in human disease.

The portion of the yeast genome that is transcribed, the 'transcriptome', has been analysed by SAGE (see p. 88). Surprisingly, several *hundred* genes were identified that were *not predicted* from analysis of the complete genome sequence. This experience is a warning about the limitations of pure sequence information.

Caenorhabditis elegans—first animal

The sequence of the nematode (worm) *Caenorhabditis elegans* was completed (with a few small gaps) at the end of 1998 by the *C. elegans* Sequencing Consortium, which fostered the release and exchange of data as it became available. The project was initiated by the development of a physical map of the genome based on the isolation and assembly of random cosmid clones. The sequence was derived from 2527 cosmids, 257 YACs, 113 fosmids and 44 PCR products.

C. elegans is famous (among scientists) for its compact complexity. The adult worm is 1 mm long, transparent, and formed of exactly 959 cells. The birth and fate of each cell follows a precise programme. It has a nervous system and exhibits behaviour. It can reproduce as a hermaphrodite (self-fertilization), which speeds genetic analysis. Genes involved in apoptosis (programmed cell death) were discovered and initially characterized in *C. elegans*. These genes have important mammalian homologues that function in development, inflammation, cancer and immunity.

Mice (Mus musculus)—key models of human disease

Mice have been intensively studied since the beginning of the 20th century because they have proven to be invaluable aids in understanding human biology. Many mouse mutants that display deep similarities with human diseases have been identified and characterized. These animals permit insights into many human diseases, such as cancer, and normal processes such as development, immunity and ageing.

Both private and public sequencing efforts are under way. The public Mouse Sequencing Consortium (MSC) is funded by pharmaceutical companies, biotechnology companies, the Wellcome Trust and the National Institutes of Health. As with the human sequencing effort, the announcement of the private Celera effort has served to galvanize the public effort. Celera reportedly has sequenced four mouse strains, providing >99% of the mouse genome. The MSC plans to sequence one strain to 95% by

2003 using a combination of map-based and shotgun approaches.

Genome modification

Transgenic animals—adding genes

> Transgenic animals have genes (transgenes) added to their genomes. This allows one to see the effect of *new, deleted* or *altered* genes.

Some questions cannot be answered with *in vitro* assays. Understanding the role of particular genes, especially those involving development or the immune system, has benefited from the ability to place new genes back into animals. Such technology may eventually allow the repair of disease-causing genes in humans.

The generation of transgenic mice followed the discovery that embryonic stem (ES) cells could be isolated from a blastocyst (an early developmental stage, preceding implantation of the fertilized egg). ES cells could be grown *in vitro* and transfected with a gene. When ES cells are mixed with fresh blastocyst cells and placed in a foster mother, they participate in the development of the mouse (Fig. 3.24). The resulting mouse is a chimera (mix) of the normal blastocyst cells and the ES cells grown *in vitro*. In some of the chimeras, the germ tissues develop from the ES cells. These animals pass on the transgene to their progeny.

There are two types of transgenes.

I *Random* insertions, where transgenes are inserted randomly anywhere the genome. Multiple copies are usually found in the transfected cell and chimera. Some of these transgenes may come under the control of different genes and be inappropriately regulated (Fig. 3.25).

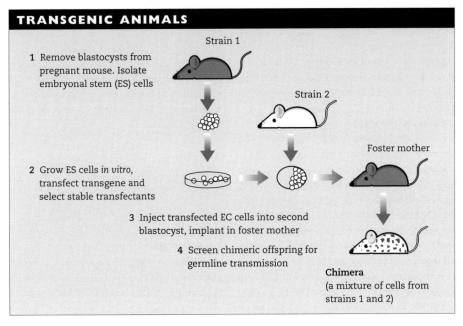

TRANSGENIC ANIMALS

Strain 1

1 Remove blastocysts from pregnant mouse. Isolate embryonal stem (ES) cells

Strain 2

Foster mother

2 Grow ES cells *in vitro*, transfect transgene and select stable transfectants

3 Inject transfected EC cells into second blastocyst, implant in foster mother

4 Screen chimeric offspring for germline transmission

Chimera
(a mixture of cells from strains 1 and 2)

Fig. 3.24 Transgenic animals—making an animal out of cells cultured *in vitro*. The cultured embryonic stem (ES) cells are added to a blastocyst and reimplanted into a foster mother. (Note that the foster mother contributes no genes to the chimera.) One formidable technical constraint has been that the ES cells can only be cultured for a limited time *in vitro* before they lose their ability to participate in the development of the animal. In some mouse strains, transgenics can be generated by adding DNA directly to the blastocyst.

RANDOM INSERTION OF A TRANSGENE

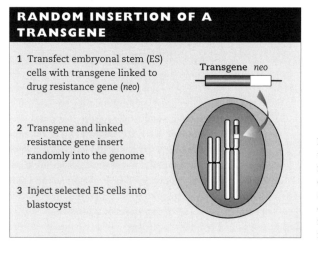

1 Transfect embryonal stem (ES) cells with transgene linked to drug resistance gene (*neo*)

2 Transgene and linked resistance gene insert randomly into the genome

3 Inject selected ES cells into blastocyst

Fig. 3.25 A transfected transgene inserts randomly into the chromosomes of ES cells in preparation for making a transgenic animal. The ES cells are selected for stable integration of the transgene into the genome.

2 *Targeted*, site-specific or homologous replacement are three names for the same event, the *replacement* of the original/normal gene with the transgene in the correct position in the genome. The frequency of homologous recombination is greatly increased by adding flanking DNA sequences that match the target region (Fig. 3.26). Nonetheless, these transgenes also insert randomly, so the cells containing the correctly targeted genes must be selected.

Random transgenics are much easier to generate than are targeted transgenics. The principal difficulty with random transgenes is the inappropriate influence of unusual genetic neighbours. This can be evaluated by analysing several independently generated transfectants. Each independent transfectant is likely to have the transgene inserted into a different site in the genome, so the effects of different neighbouring genes are averaged out.

Although the goals are to cure or prevent debilitating diseases and to understand more about life, transgenes have to date produced more sickness than health (although that tells us something about the delicacy of life). In transgenic mice, for example, overexpression of the normal cellular *myc* oncogene leads to adenocarcinomas, and expression of the viral SV40 transforming genes produces tumours.

Knockouts and knock-ins: ins and outs of gene modification

Historically, natural mutations that reduce or eliminate the activity of the encoded protein have provided the first indication of the protein's function. For example, the immune deficiency that results in elevated levels of the immunoglobulin M (hyper-IgM) provided the clue that the CD40 ligand is involved in the maturation of B cells, the producers of immunoglobulin. (Many additional examples are found in Chapter 4.)

> In 'knockout' animals, a gene is replaced with a mutant gene that does not encode the normal gene product.

Gene 'knockout' technology can provide exactly the mutant you want now, without waiting for an 'experiment of nature'. Knockout mice have already helped to define the function (or often the apparent dispensability) of many genes.

Knockout mice are a subset of *targeted transgenes*, inserted by homologous recombination, in which the target gene is deleted or interrupted by *insertional mutagenesis* (Fig. 3.26).

Remarkable genetic redundancy has been observed in many experimental systems,

GENE 'KNOCKOUT'

1 Transfect ES cells with resistance gene **flanked** by normal gene sequences and **linked** to susceptibility gene

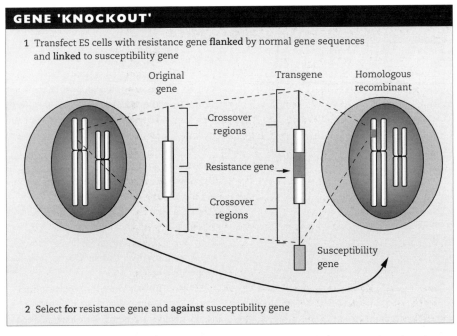

2 Select **for** resistance gene and **against** susceptibility gene

Fig. 3.26 Targeted transgenes can 'knock out' homologous genes. The resistance gene interrupts the gene that is targeted, resulting in a specific mutation of that gene. Large flanking regions encourage site-specific insertion by homologous recombination, which results in the loss of the susceptibility gene. The selected ES cells are then injected into a blastocyst. Although only one of the two genes has been mutated, mating the heterozygous offspring could breed a homozygous mouse.

where the deletion of one gene has little or no apparent effect (phenotype). This can be a huge surprise, as when myoglobin knock-out mice proved to be relatively normal. At the other extreme, some knockouts die as embryos because the deleted gene has an unexpected role in development. The most illuminating knockouts have been those in which the deleted gene is important enough to cause a problem when it is missing and the function can be inferred from the nature of the defect.

Once the knockout has demonstrated the importance of a gene, the process can be repeated to replace the defective gene with a variant gene. This process, called 'knock-in', can compare the functions of particular alleles.

Conditional knockout: Cre-Lox

If a gene is necessary for normal development, then it cannot be simply knocked out to test its function in differentiated tissues because the mouse will die before it matures. Instead, you want to knock it out *only* in the mature tissues. You can do this with the transposition system called Cre-Lox that was originally described in viruses (Fig. 3.27).

Cre is a protein enzyme that excises DNA flanked by specific DNA sequences called Lox sites. When the gene encoding the Cre protein is put under control of a tissue-specific promoter, then Cre is made only in the tissue and the target gene is deleted. One application of this system is in T cells, where the promoter for the differentiation marker CD4 can be used to express the Cre transgene in helper T cells.

CRE-LOX: REGULATED GENOMIC MODIFICATION

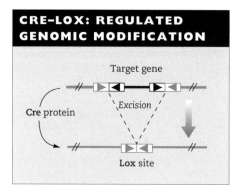

Fig. 3.27 The Cre protein mediates the excision of DNA flanked by specific Lox sequences. The expression of the Cre gene may be restricted to specific tissues. The target gene is deleted from the genome of cells in these tissues.

The promoter of the gene encoding endothelial nitric oxide synthase (eNOS), an enzyme involved in blood pressure regulation, can be used to direct Cre transgene expression in vascular endothelial cells. Alternatively, the Cre gene can be placed under control of an *inducible* promoter, which can be switched on at the desired time of development. One such promoter is the synthetic, tetracycline-regulated promoter.

Cloning animals

The manipulations of pluripotent 'stem' cells (cells that can generate an entire animal) have advanced the technology of animal cloning (Fig. 3.28). Cloning by somatic cell nuclear transfer allows the expansion of animals with desirable characteristics. This has obvious applications in propagating farm animals or transgenic animals, where yields may be increased.

Ethics

New biomedical technologies have raised new, and old, ethical questions.

• Human cloning is probably possible with modifications of those techniques that have been successful in other animals. However, experimentation in human cloning has been banned in many countries.

• Xenotransplantation is the transplantation of tissues from non-humans, such as pigs. Rejection problems are being solved by a variety of approaches, including altering the donor tissue and treating the recipient. However, there is a fear that endogenous viruses within the genomes of other species may be transferred to graft recipients. The retrovirus would be thereby 'humanized' and become a danger to all humans. A moratorium on xenotransplantation has been called for until the risks are better understood.

CLONING

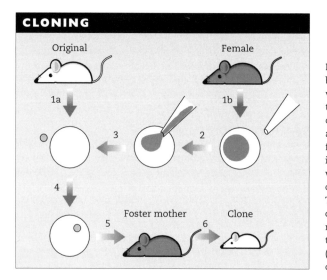

Fig. 3.28 Animals are cloned by replacing an egg nucleus with a diploid nucleus from the original. A somatic cell is obtained from the original (1a) and an egg is obtained from a female donor (1b). The nucleus is aspirated from the egg (2–3), which is fused to the somatic cell by electric shock (4). The single cell embryo is cultured for several days. The multicellular blastocyst is then transferred to a foster mother (5), which gives birth to the clone (6).

• Embryo selection can ensure that healthy children are born even to high-risk parents who are carriers for genetic disease. However, the ability to select genomes, and eventually to manipulate them, also raises the possibility of selection based on questionable traits, such as sex or appearance. These questions are similar to those raised by eugenics.

• Transgenic humans could probably be generated by inserting a gene into *germ* cells. (Gene therapy usually involves somatic cells.) In some cases, such as correcting mutations that cause human disease, this would raise few ethical questions. Altering otherwise healthy genomes, however, would raise questions of whether the risks could be justified.

• Embryonic stem cells are clearly capable of differentiating into all tissues (pluripotent). Embryonic stem cells have shown promise in trial therapies for Parkinson's disease and other diseases. 'Surplus' embryos remaining-after *in vitro* fertilizations are under consideration as sources of stem cells.

• Adult stem cells may not be fully pluripotent and they may not proliferate indefinitely. Nevertheless, they have been shown to differentiate into a wide variety of tissues. Moreover, they have the advantage of being derived from the patient, reducing infection risk and obviating immune tolerance problems. No substantive ethical questions have been raised regarding the use of adult stem cells.

Some of these questions will be resolved as the technologies are better understood. For example, recombinant DNA technology is now widely regarded as relatively safe. Originally, however, it was feared that dangerous mutant organisms could be produced in the laboratory and released into the surrounding communities, accidentally or intentionally. These fears were addressed by organizing committees that issued guidelines that are now incorporated into standard laboratory practices.

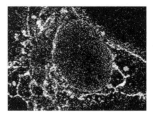

Molecular Medicine in Practice

The understanding, diagnosis and treatment of many clinical conditions have been influenced by advances in molecular medicine. These include infectious diseases (including AIDS), cancer, monogenic disorders such as cystic fibrosis, polygenic disorders such as hypertension and diabetes mellitus, and organ transplantation. This chapter deals with the effects of recently developed technologies on clinical medicine, ranging from the cloning of proteins to the cloning of mammals.

Cloning is the production of identical molecules, cells or individuals, derived from a single ancestral origin.

Biotechnology in clinical medicine

Making proteins—recombinant DNA technology

Perhaps the most widely recognized application of all recent advances in molecular medicine has been the use of recombinant DNA technology to make proteins. Once the gene for a particular protein has been cloned it can be inserted into the genome of microorganisms or cultured cells, which then produce the protein.

Recombinant DNA technology has allowed production of large quantities of pure proteins which are now in use in clinical practice. The first recombinant human protein to be used clinically was the hormone insulin. Many others have followed (Table 4.1), including growth hormone, the thrombolytic enzyme tissue-type plasminogen activator (t-PA), erythropoietin (a hormone produced in the kidney which stimulates red cell production, and is deficient in patients with renal failure), and factor VIII (the clotting factor which is deficient in haemophilia). These recombinant proteins minimize the risk of transmitting infections encountered with proteins purified from human or animal tissue, and unlike animal proteins, they are not recognized as foreign by the immune system.

The development of these products relies on considerable investment of both time and money from scientists and biotechnology companies, but the clinical, therapeutic and financial rewards are clear.

Detecting RNA, DNA and protein

Polymerase chain reaction
The polymerase chain reaction (PCR) provides a simple, fast, sensitive method of amplifying minute quantities of DNA (and RNA).

Clinical applications of PCR include:
- the detection of bacterial, fungal or viral DNA (or RNA) in clinical infections (p. 127);
- the amplification of segments of genomic DNA to look for mutations within known genes (p. 71); and
- tissue typing prior to organ transplantation (p. 131)

Table 4.1 Examples of proteins which entered clinical practice during the first decade of recombinant DNA technology (many more have followed).

RECOMBINANT PROTEINS IN CLINICAL PRACTICE

Recombinant protein	Therapeutic use	Year of product approval
Human insulin	Diabetes mellitus	1982
Human growth hormone	Growth hormone deficiency in children	1985
Interferon-α	Hairy cell leukaemia	1986
	Chronic hepatitis A and C	1992
Tissue-type plasminogen activator (t-PA)	Myocardial infarction	1987
Erythropoietin	Anaemia in chronic renal failure	1989
Granulocyte colony-stimulating factor (G-CSF)	Neutropenia following cancer chemotherapy	1991
Granulocyte–macrophage colony-stimulating factor (GM-CSF)	Myeloid reconstitution after bone marrow transplantation	1991
Factor VIII	Haemophilia A	1992

In addition the ability to amplify DNA from minute samples of tissue makes PCR an invaluable tool in forensic medicine.

Monoclonal antibodies—tools for diagnosis and treatment

Antibodies are glycoproteins which are expressed on the surface of B lymphocytes. All of the antibodies on an individual B lymphocyte have identical antigen-binding sites, which are capable of recognizing a specific antigen. When an antibody on a B lymphocyte binds to an antigen, in the presence of factors released by T helper lymphocytes, the B lymphocyte multiplies and differentiates into plasma cells which secrete antibodies bearing the same antigen-binding sites. Secreted antibodies bind to antigen, forming immune complexes which activate the complement system (see box).

Antibodies are also known as immunoglobulins. Their basic structure is shown in Fig. 4.1.

Each antibody molecule has two identical heavy chains and two identical light chains. The amino acid sequences of the N-terminal domains vary between different antibody molecules,

COMPLEMENT SYSTEM

Complement system is a series of plasma proteins which are activated sequentially. Immune complexes are a trigger for activation of this cascade of proteins, which can either directly destroy the foreign antigen or facilitate its recognition and phagocytosis by polymorphonuclear leucocytes or macrophages.

whereas the structure of the C-terminal domain is quite constant.

The N-terminal domain is known as the variable region, and is the region of the antibody that binds to antigen. Each antibody molecule has two antigen-binding sites. Most of the variation occurs in three hypervariable regions, each of which is only 6–10 amino acids long. Tremendous diversity is needed in this region to allow recognition of the enormous number of pathogens it may encounter. It has been estimated that 100 billion different antibodies can be generated by 100 billion different lymphocytes.

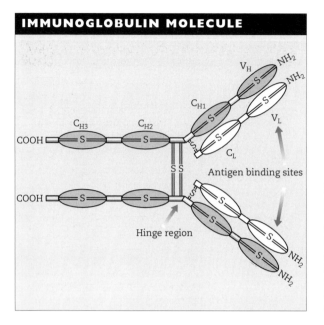

IMMUNOGLOBULIN MOLECULE

Fig. 4.1 The basic structure of an immunoglobulin molecule. The heavy chain (shaded) is made up of constant domains (C_{H1}, C_{H2}, C_{H3}) and a variable domain (V_H). The light chain has a constant domain (C_L) and variable domain (V_L). The structure is held together by disulphide bonds =S=.

The C-terminal domains of the heavy and light chains form the constant regions. The constant region of the light chain exists in two alternative forms, known as kappa (κ) and lambda (λ). Antibody molecules have either two kappa or two lambda light chains.

There are five major classes of antibody, which differ in both structure and function (Table 4.2).

The problem of how B cells are able to use their DNA to generate such an enormous diversity of antibodies caused quite a headache for immunologists, until it was discovered that the DNA encoding the different regions of an antibody molecules differs in adult B cells from that in embryo cells. It became clear that a process of programmed rearrangement occurs in the chromosomal DNA of B cells as they mature. Different rearrangements bring particular combinations of coding DNA together, accounting for the tremendous variety of antibody molecules. The process is now clear to immunologists and a headache for students.

Immunoglobulin heavy chains, lambda light chains and kappa light chains are encoded in three different genetic loci on 14q, 22q and 2p, respectively. Each region differs in its organization, although each has multiple regions encoding potential variable sites in the final antibody molecule.

In germ cells the heavy chain gene is made up of about 300 variable (V) region genes, and a series of constant (C) region genes which encode the constant regions for IgM (C_μ), IgD (C_δ), IgG3 ($C_\gamma 3$), IgG1 ($C_\gamma 1$), IgA1 ($C_\alpha 1$), IgG2 ($C_\gamma 2$), IgG4 ($C_\gamma 4$), IgE (C_ε) and IgA2 ($C_\alpha 2$). Between the V and C regions are two small coding regions, known as D and J. The D (for diversity) and J (for joining) regions each contain a number of D and J genes (Fig. 4.2).

During development of an individual B cell, a D segment is joined to a J segment, and the intervening DNA is deleted. The cell then selects one V region gene which is joined to the preformed DJ segment. The product encodes the variable region of the heavy chain, and is joined in the chromosome to all of the potential constant regions. The cell then makes either IgM, IgD, IgG, IgA or IgE by a combination of further DNA rearrangement, and the joining of the variable region domain to the

Table 4.2 Properties of human immunoglobulin classes.

FIVE MAJOR CLASSES OF ANTIBODY

Antibody class (subclasses)	Heavy chain	Amount in normal plasma	Characteristic features
IgM	μ	~10% of total	Forms large pentamers which are confined to the intravascular space. Appears early during immune response. Activates complement
IgG (IgG$_1$, IgG$_2$, IgG$_3$, IgG$_4$)	γ	Lots; ~75% of total	IgG$_1$ and IgG$_3$ efficiently activate complement. All subclasses cross the placenta
IgA (IgA1, IgA2)	α	~15% of total	Found predominantly as a dimer in mucosal secretions
IgD	δ	Very little; <1% of total	Found mainly on surface of circulating B lymphocytes
IgE	ε	Trace amounts only	Readily binds to receptors on basophils and mast cells

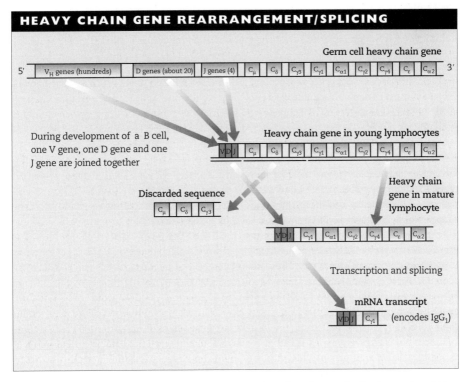

Fig. 4.2 Rearrangement and splicing of heavy chain gene in a B lymphocyte destined to produce IgG$_1$.

relevant constant region at the level of RNA processing.

A similar process occurs on different chromosomes in light chain genes, except that there is no D region in light chain genes. A V gene is joined to a J gene, and the product is joined at the RNA level to a gene encoding the constant region of kappa or lambda light chains.

The enormous diversity in antibodies synthesized by B cells results from the large number of V genes, and the way in which they can be combined with different D and J regions. Further diversity also occurs because the joining of V, D and J regions is imprecise.

Affinity maturation

B cells undergo a further process of maturation in the periphery once they encounter an antigen which they recognize. Hypermutation of the immunoglobulin V region occurs, and can lead to a dramatic improvement in antigen binding. This is followed by the selection of cells in which the mutated V region has high affinity for the antigen, a process known as affinity maturation.

Clonal nature of antibody production

The process by which antibodies are formed is known as clonal selection. Any individual produces an immense variety of B lymphocytes with different antibodies on their surface. A foreign antigen 'selects' from this population cells bearing antibodies to which it can bind. The antigen may be recognized by several different B cells bearing different antibodies, each of which may recognize a different site on the antigen, which is known as the epitope. Each cell then proliferates into a large population of cells, all of which make the same antibody. A population of identical cells that has arisen from the same ancestral cell is known as a clone, and the single antibody which is produced by such a clone is known as a monoclonal antibody.

Monoclonal antibodies can be found in the plasma of patients with myeloma. In this condition a clone of plasma cells undergoes malignant transformation, resulting in the production of a monoclonal antibody which can be detected as a discrete 'M' band on plasma protein electrophoresis. The ability to produce monoclonal antibodies in the laboratory has underpinned many achievements in molecular medicine.

Production of monoclonal antibodies

The ability to produce and use monoclonal antibodies represents one of the most important contributions to molecular biology. Monoclonal antibodies provide a precise means of identifying and testing the function of specific proteins. These include known proteins which occur in health or disease, previously unknown proteins which can then be characterized, and the products of recombinant DNA technology.

To produce a monoclonal antibody an immortal clone of B cells is produced by fusing a B cell with an immortal malignant myeloma cell (Fig. 4.3). The technology has been applied mostly to mouse antibodies, although mouse antibody genes can be modified so that the product resembles a human antibody.

In practice a mouse is injected with an antigen, and B lymphocytes which make antibodies recognize the antigen and are stimulated to grow and form clones in the spleen and bone marrow. Spleen cell suspensions from the mouse will therefore contain B cells from a number of clones which produce antibodies recognizing different sites (epitopes) on the antigen. These B-cell clones will not survive indefinitely in culture, but are made immortal by fusing them with a non-secreting myeloma cell line. The fused cells, which are known as hybridomas, produce a monoclonal antibody determined by the parent B cell, and have the immortality of the myeloma cell. Hybridomas are selected by growing the cells in medium which promotes their survival, and clones are selected by diluting the cells and assaying the supernatant for monoclonal antibodies of interest. Large-scale culture of the clones can then be used to produce quantities of pure monoclonal antibodies.

PRODUCTION OF MONOCLONAL ANTIBODIES

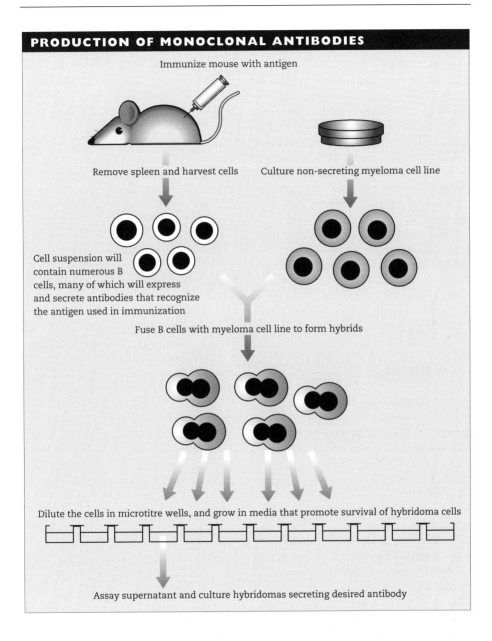

Immunize mouse with antigen

Remove spleen and harvest cells

Culture non-secreting myeloma cell line

Cell suspension will contain numerous B cells, many of which will express and secrete antibodies that recognize the antigen used in immunization

Fuse B cells with myeloma cell line to form hybrids

Dilute the cells in microtitre wells, and grow in media that promote survival of hybridoma cells

Assay supernatant and culture hybridomas secreting desired antibody

Fig. 4.3 Production of monoclonal antibodies.

Applications of monoclonal antibodies
Monoclonal antibodies have found applications in both basic science and clinical diagnosis and treatment. These are dealt with under the appropriate sections, but include:

• identification of proteins in detection assays;
• characterization of the structure and function of proteins using antibodies which specifically recognize different epitopes on a protein;
• diagnosis of infectious diseases;
• cancer diagnosis and treatment—by linking other molecules to antibodies which recognize

tumour markers, they can be used to image tumours or to target drugs against tumours;

• immunosuppression—antibodies directed against proteins expressed on lymphocytes can interfere with cell function. For example, the monoclonal antibody OKT3 that binds to the T-cell receptor has been used as an immuno-suppressant in transplantation. The usefulness of these antibodies can be limited if patients develop a human anti-mouse antibody response, and strategies to 'humanize' the constant domains of therapeutic antibodies have been developed;

• inflammatory disease—treatment with anti-bodies that neutralize the pro-inflammatory cytokine tumour necrosis factor is effective in controlling disease activity in rheumatoid arthritis and Crohn's disease (an inflammatory bowel disorder), and is likely to prove bene-ficial in other inflammatory conditions.

Genetic diseases

Inherited diseases may result from a wide spectrum of genetic abnormalities, ranging from a single base change within a gene, as in sickle cell anaemia, to the loss or addition of a complete chromosome, as in Turner syn-

TURNER AND DOWN SYNDROME

In Turner syndrome only one X chromosome is present. Affected females are short and the neck may appear webbed. Ovaries fail to develop properly leading to primary amenorrhoea (menstruation never starts). IQ is normal.

In Down syndrome an extra chromosome 21 (trisomy 21) results in the typical facial appearance (flat face, slanting eyes, small low-set ears) and simian crease (single palmar crease), together with mental retardation and an increased incidence of congenital heart disease.

drome (Fig. 4.4) and Down syndrome (Fig. 4.5), respectively.

However, the commonest human diseases are polygenic, resulting from the combined effects of multiple genes at different loci, each of which has a small but additive effect. Most of these also involve environmental factors, so that the cause is said to be multifactorial.

Impact of molecular biology on genetic diseases

Once a gene has been fully characterized, abnormalities leading to the disease associated

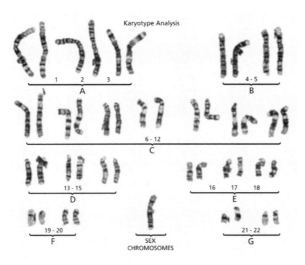

Fig. 4.4 Karyotype of Turner syndrome (XO). Karyotypes courtesy of Genetics Laboratories, Addenbrooke's Hospital, Cambridge. Chromosomes can be precisely identified by banding patterns. In addition, chromosomes can be assorted into seven groups (A to G) according to size and shape.

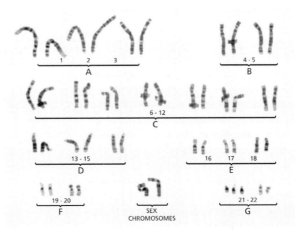

Fig. 4.5 Karyotype of Down syndrome (trisomy 21).

with it can be identified at the level of both the DNA sequences and the protein which it encodes. This often leads to an improved understanding of the disease process, and can allow detection of the abnormal gene in DNA samples from patients who have or are susceptible to the disease, carriers and the unborn fetus. The diagnosis of a genetic disorder is only useful if it is of benefit to the patient or their family. Such benefits may be obvious if there is a readily available treatment for the condition. In many cases treatments are not currently available, and the options are restricted to providing information and advice about the risk of transmitting an inherited disorder to offspring (genetic counselling) or the consideration of aborting an affected fetus.

Prenatal diagnosis

Screening for chromosomal abnormalities, such as trisomy 21 (Down syndrome), is generally available for mothers at risk due to age or a previous history of chromosomal disorders. In addition, it is now possible to screen fetal DNA for the presence of specific gene disorders.

DNA for prenatal diagnosis is usually obtained from the fetus by amniocentesis or chorionic villus sampling.

Amniocentesis is performed between 14 and 20 weeks' gestation, and involves aspiration of amniotic fluid which contains fetal cells from around the fetus using a needle passed through the abdominal wall. The fluid contains cells shed from the developing fetus, which can be used for chromosomal and DNA analysis. In addition the fluid may be assayed for components such as α-fetoprotein, which is elevated in spina bifida.

The chorion is a layer of fetal extra-embryonic tissue which spreads over and invades the uterine wall during early pregnancy. The chorion can be biopsied after the 9th week of gestation, either through the vagina and cervix or across the abdominal wall.

In specialized centres fetal blood sampling provides a source of tissue for genetic analysis. It is performed by using ultrasound guidance to sample blood from the umbilical vein of the developing fetus.

If the DNA sequence encoding the gene of interest is known, DNA from the fetus can be screened for the presence or absence of the normal gene. This usually involves developing a probe for the normal gene, and seeing if this recognizes a normal sequence in the fetal DNA, using the process of Southern blotting (see p. 48). An alternative approach is to determine whether a mutation has altered a restriction site within the gene, by looking for different-sized fragments following digestion of the region of interest with a restriction enzyme.

If the exact location and sequence of the gene is unknown the probability of a fetus carrying the gene can be determined by linkage analysis. DNA from the fetus is screened for markers, such as other genes or polymorphic microsatellite markers, which are known to be closely linked to the gene. These techniques are becoming used less frequently as more genes are identified, and direct analysis for mutations can be performed.

Any form of fetal sampling carries a risk to the fetus. These methods are usually only offered if risk factors such as advanced maternal age or a family history of a genetic disorder are present. Ultrasound and maternal blood sampling provide less invasive methods of screening for abnormalities.

Ultrasound is widely used for assessing fetal growth and development. As the resolution of ultrasound has increased it has provided a safe non-invasive method of screening for physical changes such as spina bifida, heart defects, abnormal skeletal development, cleft lip and palate, and abnormalities of the renal tract and genitals.

Maternal blood sampling has provided an important method of screening for Down syndrome. A 'triple screen' uses α-fetoprotein (AFP), unconjugated oestriol and human chorionic gonadotrophin (hCG), in combination with maternal age, weight and gestational age, to estimate the risk of Down syndrome. Low levels of AFP and unconjugated oestradiol and an elevated level of hCG increase the likelihood of the fetus having Down syndrome.

Gene therapy

The identification of genes involved in many common diseases has led to speculation that the treatment of genetic disorders by correcting the underlying abnormality through gene therapy could become a reality. Present efforts are focused on somatic gene therapy, in which defective genes are corrected in specific cells or organs rather than in egg or sperm cells, or early embryos (germline therapy).

Two approaches have been used, ex vivo and in vivo gene delivery.

In ex vivo delivery, cells are taken from a patient, the new gene is inserted, and the cells are then replaced. In vivo delivery involves targeting the gene directly to the patient's tissues, usually by infecting them with a virus which contains the new gene.

Before considering the possibility of gene therapy:

- the gene must have been cloned and sequenced so that it is fully characterized and readily available in its correct form;
- it must be possible to introduce the gene safely and efficiently into appropriate target cells; and
- the gene must be expressed in its new site.

Any of the methods used to transfect cells can be used to introduce the gene, including direct injection, calcium microprecipitation and electroporation (see p. 51). However, one of the favoured methods is to incorporate the gene into a virus, which is then used to infect the target cell. Viruses have evolved to incorporate nucleic acid into cells and induce new gene expression, often without cytotoxicity. They are thus ideally suited to achieve a high efficiency of gene transfer and expression. The most commonly used viruses are derived from murine retroviruses. Although the use of viral vectors poses potential risks because of the pathogenic nature of viruses, most of the harmful viral genes can be removed.

Viral vectors

Retroviral vectors

Retroviruses have a single-stranded RNA genome, which is converted into DNA within a cell by reverse transcriptase carried by the virus particle. The DNA is then incorporated into the host genome, where it is expressed to produce new viral RNA, together with proteins needed to form new viral particles. These are the gag, pol and env genes which code for the core proteins, the reverse transcriptase and the viral core proteins, respectively (see p. 129). Retroviruses can be prepared for gene therapy by replacing the gag, pol and env genes with the gene to be used for therapy.

One of the major advantages of retroviruses is their high efficiency of integration into the host genome, which is followed by stable expression of the introduced gene even after cell division. However, infection of non-replicating cells is poor, and the stability of the virus is adversely affected by the introduction of large gene inserts. Retroviruses are therefore best suited for the introduction of small genes into replicating cells.

Lentiviruses

Lentiviruses are a subclass of retroviruses that can infect both proliferating and non-proliferating cells, and can provide efficient transfer of genes to the central nervous system (CNS). Concerns have been expressed over their safety. These relate particularly to the risk of reversion to wild-type virus, and the potential for mutagenesis at the site of their insertion into DNA, leading to oncogenic transformation.

Adenoviruses

Adenoviruses are double-stranded DNA viruses which have been used in live viral vaccines for many years, providing a long safety record. Adenoviruses can infect non-dividing cells, but viral DNA does not integrate efficiently into the host genome, and may not be transferred to daughter cells. This raises the possibility that in tissues undergoing cell turnover, introduced DNA may be lost, and need to be reintroduced at regular intervals.

Adenoviruses are particularly attractive for use in gene therapy of respiratory disorders because of the tendency of the virus to infect cells lining the airways.

Herpes simplex virus type 1 (HSV-1)

HSV-1 is a large double-stranded DNA virus which has been extensively studied as a human pathogen. Following primary infection, usually though mucous membranes of the mouth, it lies dormant in neurones, from where it may be reactivated, often causing 'cold sores' on the lips. The neurotrophic nature of this virus makes it a candidate for gene therapy in neurological disease.

HSV-1 vectors are similar in many respects to adenovirus vectors. They can infect non-dividing cells and are not integrated into the host genome. To make room for insertion of new genetic material, DNA sequences are deleted to render them replication defective or limit their toxicity.

Adeno-associated viruses

The adeno-associated virus is a small, non-pathogenic parvovirus. It is incapable of autonomous replication, requiring coinfection with another virus (either adenovirus or herpes simplex virus). Because of its small size adenovirus-associated vectors can only accommodate inserts of less than 5 kb. Adeno-associated viruses are unique in that they integrate into a specific site on chromosome 19.

RNA viruses

RNA viruses are usually small (less than 20 kb). Many amplify and transcribe their genomes exclusively in the cytoplasm of mammalian cells, resulting in high levels of expression without the risks associated with integration into host cell DNA. Cytoplasmic expression is usually transient. This limits applications to short-term gene therapy, such as the treatment of cancer. Their role in vaccine development is also being explored.

Potential risks of viral vectors

• Viral vectors which integrate into the genome may cause DNA mutations (insertional mutagenesis).

• Recombination of the disabled viral vector with wild-type virus may lead to infectious complications.

• The virus can induce an inflammatory and immune response which may limit long-term effectiveness.

Non-viral delivery systems

Concerns over the safety and potential immunogenicity of viral gene transfer systems have led to the development of non-viral delivery systems. The simplest of these is the administration of naked DNA. Plasmid DNA (see p. 26) injected directly into muscle can be taken up and expressed by myocytes, providing a potential mechanism for the treatment of genetic diseases of skeletal muscle. This approach can also be used in vaccine development, by expressing foreign proteins to elicit a protective immune response (see *DNA vaccines*, p. 129). To improve the efficiency of gene transfer, a number of methods for encapsulating plasmid DNA have been developed. Liposomes are synthetic vesicles composed of a lipid bilayer which fuses with cell membranes. Cationic lipids and polymers can also form complexes with DNA in a way which facilitates incorporation into the cell, without the need to encapsulate the DNA. Delivery of DNA into the cell, and its transfer to the nucleus, can be further enhanced by incorporating viral components which promote cell entry or nuclear targeting.

Liposomal-mediated gene transfer has been used in human gene therapy trials of cystic fibrosis (see p. 112). Although it is less efficient than adenoviral vectors, it appears to lack the toxicity and immunogenicity reported with adenoviral vectors.

The approach adopted when considering gene therapy varies considerably, and depends on the nature of the disorder and the organ involved. The haematopoietic system, liver and skeletal muscle are among regions which are currently under investigation. Haematological disorders have provided the initial focus for gene therapy as there are already well established procedures for bone marrow transplantation. Bone marrow cells can be readily sampled, transfected and returned to the patient. In contrast, treatment of muscular dystrophy requires a different approach as correction of the defective cytoskeletal protein dystrophin requires targeting of the new gene to a large number of muscle cells, making *in vivo* gene delivery the most feasible approach.

To illustrate the diverse nature of the problems encountered when considering gene therapy, we will first consider in some detail conditions in which progress towards develop-

ing gene therapy has already been achieved. Examples of a number of genetic diseases which are currently undergoing trials of gene therapy, or likely to become targets for such therapy are then listed.

Conditions in which progress has been made towards gene therapy

Adenosine deaminase (ADA) deficiency

Adenosine deaminase (ADA) catalyses the deamination of adenosine and deoxyadenosine. Deficiency results in accumulation of deoxyadenosine and its metabolites which inhibit DNA synthesis. The gene is widely expressed in body tissues, but ADA deficiency predominantly affects lymphocyte function, and in particular appears to prevent T-lymphocyte differentiation in the thymus. This leads to varying degrees of T- and B-cell dysfunction, including neonatal onset severe combined immunodeficiency (ADA-SCID), and milder, later onset immunodeficiency. Heterozygote carriers with only 10% of ADA activity can have normal immune function.

Some patients respond to enzyme replacement therapy by intramuscular injection of ADA which has been conjugated with polyethylene glycol (PEG) to increase its half-life. Successful bone marrow transplantation cures the immunological defect, but is not available for all patients. Interestingly, results from bone marrow transplant recipients show that ADA-producing lymphoid cells appear to have a growth advantage in ADA-deficient patients. Furthermore, full immune reconstitution has been observed even if only T lymphocytes from the donor engraft.

Several features made ADA deficiency suitable for the first human gene therapy trial:
• the gene for ADA was cloned in 1983 and is relatively small with a cDNA of about 1.1 kb;
• *ex vivo* targeting of the gene to lymphocytes could be used to correct the immunological defect; and
• partial restoration of enzyme activity was predicted to be sufficient to restore normal lymphocyte function.

In 1989 the National Institutes of Health (NIH) Recombinant DNA Advisory Committee (RAC) gave approval for the first trial. A 4-year-old and a 9-year-old girl who had not fully responded to treatment with ADA-PEG were enrolled in the trial in 1990. T lymphocytes were isolated from their peripheral blood, transfected with a modified retrovirus containing the functional ADA gene, propagated in culture, and reinfused back into the girls. This procedure was repeated at approximately 2-monthly intervals for 2 years. Both children have continued with enzyme replacement therapy. Peripheral blood T-lymphocyte counts increased in both children, and tests of cell-mediated and humoral immunity increased. Measurable ADA enzyme activity increased in the younger, but not the older child. Transfected T cells could be detected in both patients 2 years after the last treatment.

In an Italian trial involving two young children transfected peripheral T lymphocytes and T-cell-depleted bone marrow cells were reinfused over a 2-year period. The peripheral T lymphocytes and bone marrow progenitor cells were transfected separately, with two similar retroviral vectors containing the functional ADA genes. The vectors were distinguishable only by different restriction sites in a non-functional region. This allowed the origin of transfected lymphocytes which survived after reinfusion to be determined. Peripheral T-lymphocyte counts, and measurements of ADA activity, demonstrated that immunity was rapidly reconstituted by transfected peripheral T lymphocytes. This population of transfected T lymphocytes declined during the year following the last treatment, but immune function was maintained for at least a year after treatment by an increase in ADA production from bone marrow-derived leucocytes and erythrocytes. However, both patients continued enzyme replacement therapy during the trial.

A neonatal trial involved three patients in whom a prenatal diagnosis of ADA deficiency had been made. CD34+ (CD stands for cluster of differentiation) bone marrow progenitor cells were harvested from umbilical cord blood, transfected with a modified retrovirus containing the functional ADA gene, and infused intravenously on the fourth day of life. Transfected leucocytes could be detected in peripheral blood and bone marrow for 18 months. However, the number of ADA-producing cells, and the level of circulating ADA activity, remained low, and all patients have been maintained on ADA-PEG replacement therapy.

Cystic fibrosis

Cystic fibrosis is the commonest life-threatening autosomal recessive disorder of Caucasians, affecting 1 in 2500 newborns. A defect in chloride secretion by epithelial cells results in the production of abnormally viscous secretions. The accumulation of thick, sticky mucus leads to obstruction of pancreatic and biliary ducts, and predisposes to recurrent chest infections. The disease results from a defect in the cystic fibrosis transmembrane conductance regulator (CFTR), a cyclic AMP-regulated chloride transporter, the gene for which was identified in 1989 by positional cloning.

Approximately 70% of mutations in the CFTR gene are caused by a 3 base pair (bp) deletion resulting in the loss of phenylalanine at position 508 in the mature protein (the ΔF508 mutation). This defect prevents the CFTR protein reaching its site of action on the apical cell membrane. The remaining 30% of defects result from a diverse range of mutations which interfere with the intracellular trafficking or function of the CFTR protein.

Conventional therapy for cystic fibrosis includes the administration of pancreatic enzymes to aid fat absorption and intensive treatment of chest infections with physiotherapy and antibiotics.

DNA released from necrotic inflammatory cells contributes to the viscosity of the sputum in cystic fibrosis. Recombinant human deoxyribonuclease (rhDNase) has been developed as a mucolytic agent.

Despite aggressive treatment of pulmonary complications patients often die of respiratory failure in early adult life. The NIH gene therapy trial for cystic fibrosis was approved in 1992. A modified adenovirus containing the CFTR gene was delivered by bronchoscopy into the lungs of four adult patients, and epithelial cell CFTR gene expression was demonstrated in all patients. However, the efficiency of transfection was low, and no patients had evidence of continued gene expression beyond 10 days after treatment. One patient who received the highest dose of adenoviral particles developed fever, hypoxia and pulmonary infiltrates which were attributed to an inflammatory reaction to the adenoviral vector. Other studies have demonstrated transient correction of the chloride transport defect through adenoviral-mediated transfection of the CFTR gene in nasal epithelium of cystic fibrosis patients. Some patients suffered from localized inflammation, and the development of an immune response against the virus may limit its effectiveness as a vector if repeated administration is necessary. Liposomal-mediated transfer of plasmid DNA containing the CFTR gene provides an alternative method of gene delivery which appears to be well tolerated, and can partially restore chloride transport when delivered into nasal and lung epithelium.

Familial hypercholesterolaemia
Familial hypercholesterolaemia is caused by mutations in the low density lipoprotein (LDL) receptor gene. Circulating LDL delivers cholesterol to tissues, where it is needed for normal membrane and steroid hormone biosynthesis. Excess LDL is cleared by the liver where it is metabolized or excreted in bile. The LDL receptor expressed on the surface of cells facilitates the uptake of LDL into tissues. Defects of the LDL receptor increase plasma cholesterol levels, and the homozygous form of familial hypercholesterolaemia is associated with markedly elevated plasma cholesterol levels and premature death from coronary artery disease. The condition responds poorly to cholesterol-lowering drugs, but liver transplantation can correct the lipid abnormalities, indicating that reconstituting normal LDL receptor expression in hepatocytes may be sufficient to treat the disease.

A gene therapy trial for familial hypercholesterolaemia involving five patients aged between 7 and 41 started in 1992. The patients underwent hepatic resection, and at the same time a catheter was placed in the portal vein. Hepatocytes were cultured from the resected liver, and transfected with a modified retrovirus containing the functional LDL receptor gene. The transfected cells were then reinfused into the liver through the portal venous catheter. All patients tolerated the process well, despite its highly invasive nature, but the response was variable. Significant and prolonged reductions in LDL cholesterol were observed in three of the five patients, but the investigators concluded that the variable response and low level of genetic reconstitution precluded further studies.

Candidate conditions for future gene therapy
Disorders in which identification of the genetic defect has improved prospects for therapy, including the above, are summarized below.

Adenosine deaminase (ADA) deficiency
Clinical features (see p. 110). ADA catalyses the deamination of adenosine and deoxyadenosine. The gene is expressed predominantly in thymus and lymphoid tissue. Deficiency results in accumulation of deoxyadenosine and its metabolites which inhibits DNA synthesis. This leads to varying degrees of T- and B-cell dysfunction, including neonatal onset severe combined immunodeficiency (ADA-SCID) and milder, later onset immunodeficiency.

Disease-related gene product. Adenosine deaminase (20q12–13).

Progress towards therapy. Long-term stable expression of the ADA gene can be achieved ex vivo in human T lymphocytes using retroviral vectors. Significant immune reconstitution has been achieved in patients following periodic infusions with ADA gene-corrected autologous T cells (see p. 111).

Adrenoleucodystrophy

Clinical features. X-linked metabolic disorder which afflicted Lorenzo Odone whose story was told in the film *Lorenzo's Oil.* Accumulation of saturated very long chain fatty acids in the brain and adrenal glands leads to progressive neurological disability and adrenal failure.

Disease-related gene product. The adrenoleucodystrophy gene (Xq28) encodes a member of the ATP-binding cassette protein transporter family, a group of proteins important for transporting molecules across cell membranes. It is not yet known how the defect leads to accumulation of very long chain fatty acids, but these substances are normally degraded in peroxisomes and the protein is found in the peroxisomal membrane.

Progress towards therapy. The adrenoleucodystrophy protein is one of a family of transporters which combine to form channels in cell membranes. The identification of these transporters in yeast cells and the development of a mouse knockout model (see p. 96) should help to define the exact role of the protein.

Adult polycystic kidney disease

Clinical features. Autosomal dominant condition in which renal failure results from progressive cystic degeneration of the kidneys.

Disease-related gene product. Approximately 85% of cases are due to a defect in *PKD1* which maps to 16p13.3 and encodes the protein polycystin 1. The gene was identified by analysis of a Portuguese family in which tuberous sclerosis (mapped in 1993 to 16p13.3) and adult polycystic kidney disease exist in different family members. A mother and daughter with adult polycystic disease (but not tuberous sclerosis) were found to have a balanced translocation between chromosomes 16 and 22, with a breakpoint on chromosome 16 at 16p13.3. The breakpoint disrupted a gene encoding a 14-kb transcript, and the identification of different mutations of that gene in other patients with adult polycystic kidney disease confirmed that it was *PKD1*. More than three-quarters of the gene is duplicated elsewhere on chromosome 16. Screening for mutations requires care to ensure that they arise in *PKD1* rather than duplicated regions.

The *PKD2* gene, responsible for most non-16p-linked polycystic kidney disease has been localized to 4q13–23.

Polycystin 1 is a large protein which spans the surface of the cell, threading in and out of the cell's membrane. Most of the protein lies outside the cell where it could interact with proteins on or around neighbouring cells, perhaps allowing cells to pass messages between each other. In contrast, the structure of the smaller polycystin 2 protein suggests that it may form ion channels in the cell's surface, and regulate the movement of molecules in and out of the cell.

Progress towards therapy. Further characterization of the underlying functional defect should help to identify potential therapies.

Alpha 1-antitrypsin deficiency

Clinical features. Alpha 1-antitrypsin (α_1-antitrypsin) is the major serine-proteinase inhibitor present in blood. (Serine-proteinases are a group of proteolytic enzymes, including trypsin, chymotrypsin and elastase, in which the amino acid serine forms part of the active enzyme site.) Deficiency of α_1-antitrypsin predisposes individuals to liver disease in childhood, and lung disease in adult life.

Disease-related gene product. Alpha 1-antitrypsin (14q) which normally encodes the 'M' subtype of the protein. Two common mutations give rise to 'S' and 'Z' variants of α_1-antitrypsin, in which abnormal folding of the protein alters both its structure (favouring formation of polymers which may become deposited in liver) and function.

Progress towards therapy. Retroviral-mediated transfer of the normal α_1-antitrypsin gene into cultured mammalian cells has been achieved. However, if the disease is in part related to the presence of the abnormal protein, transfer of the normal gene into patients may not correct the pathology completely.

Cystic fibrosis
Clinical features (see p. 111). Autosomal recessive disorder of glandular tissue resulting in the production of abnormally thick secretions. Predominantly affects the respiratory tract and pancreas.

Disease-related gene product. Cystic fibrosis is caused by mutations of the cystic fibrosis transmembrane conductance regulator (CFTR) gene (*CFTR*) (7q31.2). CFTR functions as a cAMP-regulated chloride channel on the apical surface of airway and other epithelial cells.

Progress towards therapy. Transfer of the normal *CFTR* gene to cystic fibrosis epithelial cells *in vitro* corrects the defective chloride channel regulation. The feasibility of using an adenovirus vector to transfer and express CFTR cDNA in the respiratory epithelium of patients with cystic fibrosis has been demonstrated. This approach may therefore provide a strategy for correcting the cystic fibrosis phenotype (see p. 112).

di George syndrome
Clinical features. Many of the features can be accounted for by a disturbed migration of embryonic cells to form tissues in the head and neck (specifically the migration of the cervical neural crest into the derivatives of the pharyngeal arches and pouches). Underdevelopment of the parathyroid glands leads to a loss of parathyroid hormone and hypocalcaemia, thymic hypoplasia interferes with T-cell maturation causing immunodeficiency, and there

are often defects in the major blood vessels arising from the heart and abnormal facial features.

Disease-related gene product. di George syndrome is caused by a deletion of the *DGS* region on chromosome 22, produced by an error in recombination at meiosis. Several genes from the region of 22q11 are lost.

Progress towards therapy. The clinical picture varies according to the amount of genetic material lost. At present different therapies are directed towards the variable phenotype which has been given the acronym CATCH 22 for cardiac, abnormal facies, thymic hypoplasia, cleft palate, hypocalcaemia and 22nd chromosome.

Duchenne muscular dystrophy
Clinical features. X-linked recessive disorder leading to progressive skeletal and cardiac muscle dysfunction in children.

Disease-related gene product. The cytoskeletal protein dystrophin (Xp21.2) is either abnormal or absent. In Becker's muscular dystrophy a milder form of muscular dystrophy is caused by mutations of the dystrophin gene resulting in partially functional dystrophin protein which is reduced in amount or size.

Progress towards therapy. Problems are presented by the large number of affected muscle cells which need to be targeted, and the large size of the dystrophin gene (over 2 million bp), which is beyond the capacity of retroviral vectors. Truncated forms of the dystrophin gene encoding smaller, yet functional, proteins (dystrophin minigenes) have been produced. This raises the possibility of gene transfer using viral vectors.

Familial hypercholesterolaemia
Clinical features. A deficiency of the receptor for low density lipoprotein (LDL) results in hypercholesterolaemia (severe in the homozygous form, less marked in heterozygotes)

leading to atherosclerosis. Patients die prematurely, usually from myocardial infarction.

Disease-related gene product. LDL receptor (19p).

Progress towards therapy. LDL is processed in the liver, making hepatocytes the principal target for gene therapy. Replication-defective recombinant adenoviruses containing the LDL receptor gene have been expressed *ex vivo* in cultured hepatocytes from patients with LDL receptor deficiency. Preliminary reports indicate that cholesterol levels can fall following insertion of infected hepatocytes into the liver via the portal vein (see p. 112).

Fragile X syndrome
Clinical features. X-linked mental retardation is associated with tall stature and a characteristic facial appearance.

Disease-related gene product. The genetic defect is an expansion of a triplet repeat (CGG) in a gene of unknown function near the end of the long arm of the X chromosome (Xq27). The chromosome is constricted at this site, with partial detachment of the distal portion.

Progress towards therapy. Although the function of the gene is currently unknown, identification of the genetic defect offers the opportunity to detect female carriers, in addition to aiding prenatal diagnosis.

Friedreich's ataxia
Clinical features. An autosomal recessive disorder characterized by progressive loss of coordination (ataxia) and enlargement of the heart.

Disease-related gene product. Frataxin (9q13–21) is a mitochondrial protein of unknown function.

Progress towards therapy. Frataxin has homology to a yeast protein (YFH1). Study of this protein, which is involved in control of iron levels

and respiratory function, may help define the role of frataxin.

Familial Mediterranean fever
Clinical features. An autosomal recessive disorder characterized by recurrent episodes of fever and peritonitis, an inflammation of the peritoneal membrane which lines the abdominal cavity. It is commonest in non-Ashkenazi Jews, Armenian Arabs and Turks, and as many as 1 in 5 of these populations may carry the gene.

Disease-related gene product. The familial Mediterranean fever gene (16p13.3) encodes the protein marenostrin, also known as pyrin. The gene is expressed in white blood cells and is thought to promote inactivation of a chemotactic factor (probably the complement factor C5a).

Progress towards therapy. Identification of the gene mutations should allow development of a simple diagnostic test. Characterization of the protein should improve understanding of this, and other inflammatory conditions, and help identify environmental triggers that can lead to attacks.

Gaucher's disease
Clinical features. Autosomal recessive lysosomal storage disorder in which the sphingolipid glucocerebroside accumulates in the liver, spleen and bone marrow. Low white and red cell counts, enlargement of the liver and spleen and skeletal deformities occur.

Disease-related gene product. Glucocerebridase (1q21), which metabolizes glucocerebroside.

Progress towards therapy. In 1991 intravenous infusion of a modified form of the glucocerebridase enzyme became available as a form of enzyme replacement therapy. Retroviral-mediated transfer of the human glucocerebridase into cultured Gaucher bone marrow has been reported, raising the prospect of introducing transduced haematopoietic stem cells into patients.

Haemochromatosis
Clinical features. An autosomal recessive disorder in which there is excess iron absorption and deposition, chiefly in the liver, pancreas, heart, synovial membranes and endocrine glands.

Disease-related gene product. HFE (6p21.3) is a member of the major histocompatibility complex class I-like family, which complexes with the transferrin receptor, lowering its affinity for transferrin.

Progress towards therapy. Identification of the genetic defect may facilitate the introduction of screening programmes. Regular venesection provides an effective treatment.

Haemoglobinopathies
Clinical features. Normal adult haemoglobin is made up of two polypeptide chains, the α and β chains, which are folded such that each chain can hold an oxygen-binding haem molecule. The haemoglobinopathies are a diverse group of autosomal recessive disorders of haemoglobin synthesis which include sickle cell anaemia (abnormal β-chain synthesis) and the thalassaemias (deficient or absent α- or β-chain synthesis). Together they form the commonest group of single gene disorders in the world population.

Disease-related gene products. Genes encoding five different β-globin chains and three different α-globin chains are expressed in a precisely regulated manner during different stages of development. For example, during fetal life the two β-globin variants called γ-globin combine with two α-globin chains to give rise to fetal haemoglobin. During adult life the β-globin variants themselves combine with α-globin chains to form adult haemoglobin. The five β-globin chain genes are clustered on chromosome 11, whereas the α-globin chain genes occur together on chromosome 16. Numerous different mutations in the α-globin and β-globin genes have been described, which give rise to α or β thalassaemia, respectively. Sickle

cell anaemia is caused by a point mutation, which involves substitution of T for A in the second nucleotide of the sixth codon changing the sixth amino acid from glutamine to valine (see p. 65).

Progress towards therapy. Globin genes are highly expressed only in erythroid cells in a tightly regulated manner. Attempts to produce high-level regulated expression of globin genes have so far been unsuccessful.

Haemophilia
Clinical features. Sex-linked recessive clotting disorder in which patients suffer mainly from spontaneous bleeding into joints and soft tissues, and excessive bleeding in response to trauma or surgery.

Disease-related gene product. Haemophilia A (classical haemophilia) or haemophilia B (Christmas disease) result from defects in clotting factor VIII (Xq28) or factor IX (Xq27), respectively.

Progress towards therapy. The lack of requirement for tissue-specific expression or precise regulation of the deficient factors (small amounts have significant clinical benefits and large amounts do not appear harmful), make haemophilia an excellent candidate for gene therapy. Implantation of autologous skin fibroblasts, transduced with a retroviral vector encoding factor IX, have been reported to partially correct the haemorrhagic tendency in two Chinese patients with haemophilia B.

Huntington's disease
Clinical features. Progressive dementia and involuntary movements (chorea) in middle age. Inheritance is autosomal dominant, although the disease is late and variable in its presentation.

Disease-related gene product. The Huntington's disease gene (4p16.3) contains an expanded CAG trinucleotide repeat. The gene has been denoted *IT15*, and the protein it encodes huntingtin.

Progress towards therapy. The gene encodes a novel protein of currently unknown function. Identification of the genetic mutation increases the precision of genetic testing. However, pre-symptomatic testing for Huntington's disease must be approached with great care because of the implications of a positive test for the patient and family.

Leucocyte adhesion deficiency
Clinical features. Autosomal recessive disorder characterized by recurrent bacterial infections, impaired wound healing and impaired pus formation.

Disease-related gene product. CD18 gene (21) encodes a subunit of the leucocyte function-associated antigen (LFA-1). LFA-1 interacts with another cell surface protein, intercellular adhesion molecule 1 (ICAM-1), which is expressed at high levels in inflamed tissues.

Progress towards therapy. Bone marrow cells from CD18-deficient patients infected with a retrovirus encoding the CD18 gene express CD18 in long-term culture.

Marfan's syndrome
Clinical features. An autosomal dominant disorder in which affected individuals are tall with disproportionately long limbs, and have a tendency to cardiac abnormalities (prolapse of the mitral valve and dilatation of the aortic root), and dislocation of the lens of the eye.

Disease-related gene product. The *FBN1* gene (15q21.1) encodes fibrillin 1, a major component of the microfibrils that determine the architecture of the extracellular matrix in connective tissue.

Progress towards therapy. As the mutant protein exerts a dominant negative effect (see box above) therapies have to be directed towards suppression of the expression of the mutated gene. Ribozymes (catalytic RNA molecules,

DOMINANT NEGATIVE EFFECT

A mutant molecule exerts a dominant negative effect when it interferes with the function of its normal counterpart.

Fig. 4.6 and see also p. 23) have been used to downregulate production of fibrillin 1 in cultured dermal fibroblasts.

The hammerhead ribozyme can be designed to cleave certain RNA molecules. This provides the opportunity for genetically engineered ribozyme genes to be transfected into cells where the expressed ribozyme can target and destroy specific RNA molecules.

Mucopolysaccharidoses
Hurler syndrome—type I

Clinical features. An autosomal recessive disease in which tissue deposition of mucopolysaccharides is associated with coarse facial features, clouding of the cornea, short stature and progressive mental retardation.

Disease-related gene product. There is deficiency of the enzyme α-L-iduronidase (4p16.3).

Hunter syndrome—type II

Clinical features. This sex-linked recessive form is generally less severe, and the corneas are clear.

Disease-related gene product. There is deficiency of iduronate 2-sulphatase (Xq28).

Progress towards therapy. Untreated Hurler syndrome usually leads to death in the second decade, whilst patients with Hunter syndrome typically survive into the third decade. Enzyme activity has been restored in lymphoblastoid cells from patients with Hunter syndrome which have been transduced with a retroviral vector containing the iduronate 2-sulphatase gene.

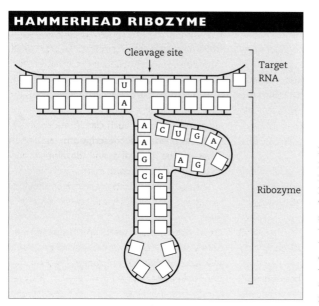

Fig. 4.6 Ribozymes are naturally occurring RNA molecules that cleave target RNA molecules at specific sites. The ribozyme has a three-stemmed structure in which two of the stems bind to the target RNA. The cleavage site contains the sequence XUY, where X is any base, U is uracil and Y is any base except guanine.

Myotonic dystrophy

Clinical features. Progressive muscle weakness in which there is continued contraction of muscles after cessation of voluntary effort (myotonia). The disorder is autosomal dominant and may be associated with cataracts, frontal baldness, mild intellectual impairment and cardiomyopathy.

Disease-related gene product. There is expansion of a CTG repeat in the 3' untranslated region of the myotonin protein kinase gene (19q13.3).

Progress towards therapy. Identification of the genetic defect has increased both the potential for screening and our understanding of the disease. The degree of expansion correlates with the severity of the disease, and anticipation is characteristic (increasing severity of the disease in successive generations due to progressive expansion of the repetitive unit).

Phenylketonuria

Clinical features. An autosomal recessive disorder in which increased blood levels of L-phenylalanine leads to mental retardation, and hypopigmentation of the skin and hair.

Disease-related gene product. Phenylalanine hydroxylase (12q22–24) converts the amino acid phenylalanine to tyrosine. Mutations in both copies of the gene lead to a build-up of toxic levels of phenylalanine.

Progress towards therapy. Phenylketonuria was the first condition for which mass screening became available. The increased phenylalanine level is detected by the Guthrie bacterial inhibition assay performed on a dried blood spot obtained by pricking the heel of neonates. With careful supervision of a phenylalanine-free diet normal development occurs. Phenylalanine hydroxylase activity has been restored in deficient mice using an adenoviral vector.

Wilson's disease (hepatolenticular degeneration)

Clinical features. An autosomal disorder of copper metabolism characterized by toxic copper deposition in the liver and brain.

Disease-related gene product. ATPase, copper-transporting, β polypeptide (ATP7B; 13q14.2–21).

Progress towards therapy. The introduction of functional ATP7B protein by adenoviral gene delivery is being investigated as a possible thera-peutic approach.

Wiskott–Aldrich syndrome

Clinical features. An X-linked disease charac-terized by eczema, thrombocytopenia and immunological defects in affected males. Female heterozygote carriers inactivate their X chro-mosome in blood cells, but not cells of other lineages.

Disease-related gene product. The Wiskott–Aldrich syndrome protein (WASP) (Xp11) interacts with a large number of lipids or other proteins involved in the regulation of signal transduction and cytoskeletal organization.

Progress towards therapy. At present bone mar-row transplantation is the treatment of choice for severe cases. Gene therapy to restore expression of normal WASP in haemopoietic stem cells provides a potentially attractive treatment option.

These examples make it clear that, although enthusiasm for pursuing options for gene therapy remains, the optimism of the last two decades that gene therapy could relieve the suffering of many patients with monogenic disorders has not yet been fulfilled. For many diseases a genetic cure remains a distant aspira-tion. Furthermore, concerns over the safety of gene therapy have been raised by a number of deaths occurring in patients in the USA, leading to a review of the process for reporting adverse events.

Polygenic disorders

Attention has now turned to the impact of molecular medicine on complex traits such as diabetes, hypertension and Alzheimer's dis-ease. The identification of genes involved in polygenic disorders may allow classification of common diseases according to the underly-ing genetic defects. Such classifications should improve phenotypic descriptions, and allow drugs to be designed and developed with specific genetic defects in mind. Available treat-ments could be tailored to individuals, select-ing drugs according to genetic abnormalities.

Unravelling the genetics of polygenic disorders

The nature of these diseases inevitably makes their genetic analysis complex. However advances in physical mapping of the genome have allowed identification of different suscep-tibility genes which are likely to be involved in the development of the same disease.

Three principal strategies have been used to identify susceptibility genes in polygenic disorders.

1 Linkage analysis tests for segregation of traits with genetic markers beyond that expected by chance in families, and is applied to affected sib-lings or relative pairs to increase the power of detection.

2 In association studies the comparison is between unrelated cases and controls.

3 Candidate genes can be directly analysed for mutations.

Candidate genes are genes which might be expected to be involved in the development of

REGULATING GENE THERAPY

In many countries gene therapy is overseen by both local and national regulatory bodies. In the USA the Director of the National Institutes of Health (NIH) approves gene therapy proposals. In making decisions the Director seeks advice from the Recombinant DNA Advisory Committee (RAC), which was established in 1974 to develop recommendations for the regulation of recombinant DNA research. In the UK the 1992 report of the Committee on the Ethics of Gene Therapy (Clothier Committee) recommended that gene therapy should be limited to life-threatening diseases or disorders. The Gene Therapy Advisory Committee (GTAC) was established in 1993 to oversee and implement its recommendations.

PHARMACOGENOMICS

Pharmacogenomics involves the application of the technologies involved in the discovery of genes to the design and development of drugs. It may serve to predict drug efficacy and the likelihood of side-effects, and to tailor the use of drugs for specific genetically defined subgroups of patients.

a multifactorial disease. For example, the genes involved in lipid metabolism are important candidates in trying to understand the polygenic inheritance of cardiovascular disease.

Consideration of recent advances in the mapping of loci for diabetes mellitus and hypertension highlights both the achievements, and the potential difficulties, in unravelling the complexities of polygenic diseases.

Diabetes mellitus

Insulin-dependent diabetes mellitus (IDDM; type I diabetes) is an autoimmune disorder in which the insulin-producing β cells of the pancreas are destroyed. It tends to occur in children and young adults. The identical twin of an IDDM patient has a 30–50% chance of developing the disease, implying that both genetic and environmental factors are involved.

Two chromosome regions have been established as being associated with, and linked to, IDDM: the major histocompatibility complex (MHC) class II region (designated *IDDM1*; 6p21) and the insulin gene region (*IDDM2*; 11p15). Genes at other loci are likely to be important, and IDMM was the first complex genetic disorder to be studied by genome-wide screening of affected sibling pairs. Several other loci have been identified by genome scanning, although different research groups have reported apparently conflicting results. However, it is likely that a consensus will emerge in the near future.

Non-insulin-dependent diabetes mellitus (NIDDM; type 2 diabetes) occurs in middle or old age. It is characterized by a resistance in tissues to the actions of insulin that is not adequately compensated for by an increase in insulin production in the pancreas. Genetically and clinically it is a heterogeneous disorder, but suceptibility genes are starting to be identified. The identification of such genes has been aided by studies of an early-onset form of type 2 diabetes known as maturity-onset diabetes of the young (MODY). MODY has an autosomal dominant inheritance, with different genetic defects being identified in different pedigrees. Mutations in the gene for insulin, the genes for insulin-processing enzymes, and the gene for the insulin receptor have all been detected. For example, a defect in the insulin promoter factor I gene has been implicated as a cause of maturity-onset diabetes of the young (*MODY4*), and identified as a significant risk factor for type 2 diabetes.

Hypertension

The identification of susceptibility loci in hypertension has proved more challenging. Blood pressure levels show strong familial aggregation which cannot be accounted for by shared environment alone. An individual is about twice as likely to develop hypertension if they have a hypertensive sibling. Rare monogenic forms of hypertension have been identified, but in the majority of patients diverse genetic and environmental factors contribute to hypertension. In all cases understanding the physiological mechanisms involved in blood pressure control provides a basis for searching for responsible genes.

Monogenic forms of hypertension

Liddle's syndrome is an autosomal dominant disorder caused by a defect in either the β or γ subunits of a sodium channel found in epithelial cells, which are encoded by genes on chromosome 16. Premature truncation of either subunit (different pedigrees exist) causes constitutive activation of the channel, increasing sodium reabsorption by the tubules of the kidney. The result is salt-sensitive hypertension, associated with low plasma potassium, and low levels of renin and aldosterone.

Apparent mineralocorticoid excess results from mutations in the gene encoding the

PHYSIOLOGY OF BLOOD PRESSURE CONTROL

Renin–angiotensin–aldosterone system
A number of factors, including hypotension, hypovolaemia and hyponatraemia, stimulate renin release from the juxtaglomerular apparatus in the kidney. Renin converts angiotensinogen to angiotensin I, which is then converted by angiotensin-converting enzyme (ACE) to angiotensin II. Angiotensin II causes arteriolar vasoconstriction, activation of the sympathetic nervous system, and secretion of the mineralocorticoid aldosterone, which promotes salt reabsorption and potassium secretion in the collecting ducts of the kidney.

Endothelins are a family of structurally related 21 amino acid peptides and the most potent vasoconstrictors known. At least three different isoforms exist. Endothelin 1 (ET-1) is the predominant peptide generated by vascular endothelial cells.

Nitric oxide (NO, originally named endothelial-derived relaxing factor) is produced by oxidation of the guanidine-nitrogen terminal of L-arginine, forming NO and citrulline. Production of NO is regulated via activity of NO synthase, a predominantly cytosolic calcium–calmodulin-requiring enzyme which is similar in structure to cytochrome P450 enzymes.

enzyme 11β-hydroxysteroid dehydrogenase, which is involved in metabolism of the steroid cortisol. Cortisol interacts with the mineralocorticoid receptor with a similar affinity to aldosterone. In the kidney the enzyme is expressed in tubules in a similar distribution to the mineralocorticoid receptor. It may thus reduce local concentrations of cortisol in the region of the mineralocorticoid receptor, leaving aldosterone to exert the predominant influence on this receptor. However, if the enzyme is defective, normal circulating levels of cortisol can produce a marked mineralocorticoid effect. The result is early-onset hypertension with the features of mineralocorticoid excess, but very low plasma aldosterone levels.

In glucocorticoid-remediable aldosteronism, hypertension is associated with excessive secretion of aldosterone which is under the control of adrenocorticotrophic hormone (ACTH) rather than angiotensin II. This is because the disease is caused by unequal crossing over during meiosis of the genes for 11β-hydroxylase and aldosterone synthase, which are close to each other on chromosome 8. This produces a novel chimeric gene, in which the coding sequence of the aldosterone synthase gene contains the regulatory sequence of 11β-hydroxylase, and is regulated by ACTH as if it were a cortisol-synthesizing gene.

Essential hypertension
These monogenic causes of hypertension are fascinating experiments of nature, but very rare. It is unclear to what extent mutations in these, and other genes which influence blood pressure, may contribute to the development of high blood pressure in the general population. Variations in the gene for angiotensinogen, which forms the substrate for renin, have been linked to hypertension in a number of studies. The aldosterone synthase gene and a region close to the epithelial sodium channel gene have also been implicated. However, other results suggest that polymorphisms in neither renin, angiotensin-converting enzyme nor nitric oxide synthase genes, the products of all of which would be expected to influence blood pressure, contribute to human hypertension.

Cardiovascular disease
Unravelling the genetic effects predisposing to cardiovascular disease is even more complex. Polygenic disorders such as hypertension and lipid abnormalities, and environmental effects such as cigarette smoking, all contribute to the development of atherosclerosis. However, advances in genetics may still prove useful in therapy. A number of angiogenic growth factors which promote formation of new blood vessels have been identified. Vascular endothelial

cell growth factor (VEGF) promotes proliferation and migration of endothelial cells lining blood vessels. Delivery of VEGF to sites of ischaemia, either as a recombinant protein or through gene transfer in the form of naked plasmid DNA, may facilitate revascularization.

Alzheimer's disease

Alzheimer's disease is characterized pathologically by degeneration of neurones in the brain, particularly affecting the cerebral cortex and hippocampus. Typically fragments of a large membrane protein (β-amyloid precursor protein) form extracellular deposits which fold into sheets known as β-amyloid. Inside cells 'tangled' tau proteins can be found.

Three genes have been identified in which autosomal dominant, highly penetrant mutations are associated with the early-onset familial form of Alzheimer's disease. These are the β-amyloid precursor protein (APP) gene on chromosome 21, presenilin 1 (PS1) on chromosome 14 and presenilin 2 (PS2) on chromosome 1. However, less than 2% of Alzheimer's disease patients are thought to carry one of these highly penetrant mutations associated with the disease. Inheritance of the E4 allele of the apolipoprotein E (ApoE) gene (APOE) is a risk factor for late-onset forms of the disease.

The identification of genes associated with Alzheimer's disease has provoked a debate concerning the value of genetic testing for the condition. Commercial tests are available for PS1 mutations and APOE alleles, but no interventions have been proven to prevent or delay the onset of Alzheimer's disease. Current recommendations are that whilst testing for highly penetrant mutations such as PS1 may be appropriate for adults, testing for susceptibility genes such as APOE should not be encouraged.

Cancer

Cancer usually arises as a result of acquired genetic changes. Environmental factors which can damage DNA, including radiation, viruses and certain chemicals (see p. 64), are therefore important and in some cases the susceptibility to such changes is inherited. A number of genes which are important in the development of tumours have been identified. It seems likely that several different genetic alterations are necessary to produce most human cancers.

Oncogenes

Retroviruses transcribe their RNA genome into DNA, which then becomes inserted into the host genome. Certain retroviruses can cause tumours in animals, and many of these tumour viruses contain genes which are capable of inducing malignant transformation in cells. These genes are called *viral oncogenes* or *v-onc* genes. Sequences that are homologous to *v-onc* genes are normally found in the genome of all vertebrate species. Thus each viral oncogene which has been identified has a normal cellular counterpart in the human genome, which is known as a cellular oncogene (*c-onc* gene) or proto-oncogene.

There are now numerous examples of these cellular oncogenes and they each have important regulatory functions in normal cell division and differentiation.

- *v-fos* causes osteosarcoma in mice.
- *c-fos*, a homologous sequence on the long arm of chromosome 14, encodes a protein which binds to DNA and regulates the expression of a number of genes.
- *v-erb-B* causes erythroblastosis in chickens.
- *c-erb-B* on the short arm of chromosome 7 encodes a truncated form of the receptor for epidermal growth factor, which appears to signal even in the absence of the growth factor.
- The *ras* family of retrovirus oncogenes cause sarcoma in the rat. Homologous sequences in the human genome encode GTP-binding proteins which are involved in cell signalling.

Oncogenes are therefore normal cellular genes which encode proteins involved in normal cell growth and division.

Tumour suppressor genes

Another group of genes involved in the development of cancer are tumour suppressor genes or *antioncogenes*. The presence of these genes in normal cells is thought to suppress the development of tumours. Mutation of the gene results in loss of suppression, favouring malignant transformation. Examples are the p53 gene and the retinoblastoma gene (see p. 125). The p53 gene, on the short arm of chromosome 17, encodes a protein of molecular weight 53 kDa. p53 is a transcription factor that can activate a wide range of genes involved in cell cycle arrest, induction of apoptosis and DNA repair. The cellular level of p53 protein increases dramatically in response to agents that damage DNA. One mechanism by which p53 regulates cell proliferation is by induction of p21, a cyclin-dependent kinase inhibitor which promotes growth arrest.

Normal p53 function can be disrupted by mutation of the gene, and also by the binding of viral proteins or cellular oncogenes to the p53 protein. For example the human papillomavirus E6 oncoprotein promotes proteosomal degradation of p53. In ataxia telangiectasia an inherited defect leads to defective post-translational modification of p53 (see p. 124).

How do oncogenes cause cancer?

Cancers occur when mutations occur in oncogenes such that their normal function of regulating cell growth, proliferation and death is disrupted. This can occur in a number of ways. Deletion of a tumour suppressor gene results in the loss of its function, and mutations within a gene may lead to production of an abnormal protein product. Gene expression may be increased by amplification of the gene so that it is present in multiple copies, whereas the chromosome breakage involved in translocations may disrupt the oncogene or bring it under the control of different promoter regions.

A number of consistent chromosomal translocations have been described in human malign-ancies, implying the involvement of oncogenes and leading to their identification.

Burkitt's lymphoma

In the majority of patients with this lymphoid tumour there is a translocation between chromosomes 8 and 14. This results in the *c-myc* gene (8q34), which is an important regulator of cell growth and cell death, being juxtaposed to the immunoglobulin heavy chain locus (14q32), thereby activating the oncogene.

Philadelphia chromosome

Reciprocal exchange of chromosomal material between chromosomes 9 and 22 gives rise to the Philadelphia chromosome in the malignant cells of patients with chronic myeloid leukaemia. The rearrangement results in the translocation of the *bcr* (breakpoint cluster region) gene (22q11) adjacent to *c-abl* (9q34), resulting in a fusion gene, and the subsequent expression of the BCR-ABL fusion protein which is involved in the malignant transformation of myeloid cells.

Too much growing or not enough dying?

The precise cellular mechanisms by which genetic alterations cause cancer are at present unknown. Recent attention has challenged the concept that cancer arises due to the abnormal proliferation of cells, and focused on the idea that malignant cells escape the normal process by which cells die.

PROTEASOME

Proteasomes are large proteases, composed of multiple subunits, that recognize, unfold and digest proteins that have been labelled for degradation, by attachment of specific markers which are usually ubiquitin molecules.

The lifespan of cells is normally controlled by a physiological process of programmed cell death, known as apoptosis.

Apoptosis is characterized by the condensation of cytoplasm and chromatin, and the fragmentation of nuclear DNA such that it appears as a 'ladder' of different-sized fragments when run on a gel. The cells disintegrate into apoptotic bodies, and are rapidly eaten by neighbouring cells.

The development and progression of certain malignancies may result from the inability of cells to die, and the characterization of genes involved in apoptosis (see box above) has provided insights into the molecular mechanisms of oncogenesis. Furthermore, it is becoming increasingly clear that many cytotoxic drugs used in the chemotherapy of cancer work by inducing apoptosis in tumour cells.

The c-myc-encoded protein is a DNA-binding transcription factor that paradoxically can induce both proliferation and apoptosis in cells. Whether a cell grows or dies in response to c-myc is likely to depend on the availability of other critical factors. For example the growth factor IGF-1 (insulin-like growth factor 1) suppresses c-myc-induced apoptosis, whereas cytotoxic drugs promote apoptosis. Deregulation of c-myc expression appears to be fundamental to the development of a number of malignancies.

The bcl-2 oncogene (located on 18q21) encodes a protein that localizes to the mitochondrial membrane, and has also been detected in the nuclear envelope. The bcl-2-encoded protein blocks apoptosis and promotes cell survival.

Evidence for a role of bcl-2 in carcinogenesis comes from genetic studies of patients with tumours of the lymphoid system. Reciprocal translocation between the long arms of chromosomes 14 and 18 is seen in 85% of patients with follicular lymphoma. In this translocation the bcl-2 gene is juxtaposed to the immunoglobulin heavy chain gene, resulting in greatly enhanced expression of the bcl-2 protein.

Familial cancer

Sometimes the development of cancer depends on a mutation occurring during life in a particular form of a gene, which has itself been inherited. Most familial cancers involve defects in tumour suppressor genes. Understanding the disease mechanisms provides valuable insights into the role of these genes.

Ataxia telangiectasia

Clinical features. An autosomal recessive disorder characterized by progressive loss of coordination (ataxia) and dilatation of small blood vessels, particularly in the eye (ocular telangiectasia). Patients also suffer from immunodeficiency, chromosomal instability, hypersensitivity to ionizing radiation and a predisposition to cancer.

Disease-related gene product. The product of the *ATM* (ataxia telangiectasia mutated) gene (11q23.1) is a kinase that activates p53 (see p. 123) by addition of a phosphate group to serine residue 15. Molecular analysis of the disorder has provided valuable insights into the cellular response and cancer risk associated with radiation exposure.

Breast cancer

Clinical features. About 5% of cases of breast cancer are due to inheritance of highly penetrant dominant susceptibility genes.

Disease-related genes. Mutations in the *BRCA1* or the *BRCA2* genes account for the majority of cases of hereditary breast cancer.

BRCA1 (17q21) encodes a nuclear protein of 1863 amino acids which contains a RING finger domain (see box), and a tandemly repeated BRCT motif thought to be involved in cell cycle regulation. BRCA1 interacts with the protein Rad51, which has been identified in yeast as a major regulator of DNA repair and recombination. Within the cell nucleus these proteins colocalize in a distribution which is influenced by cell cycle and agents which damage DNA.

BRCA2 (13q12.3) is also a nuclear protein that can interact with Rad51, and has domains that can act as transcriptional regulators.

RING FINGER

The RING finger motif is a specialized zinc finger domain (see p. 19) found in many transcriptional regulatory proteins.

The identification of susceptibility genes now allows genetic testing for predisposition to breast cancer. This raises a number of ethical issues, and careful counselling must precede any decision to screen for mutations. Testing will allow reassurance for women who have not inherited a mutated gene, but the identification of women at risk has profound psychological implications for the patient, and raises difficult issues regarding the appropriate prophylactic treatment.

Colon cancer

Clinical features. Between 5 and 15% of colon cancers are thought to be hereditary.

Disease-related genes. MLH1 (mutL (E. coli) homologue 1; 3p21.3) and MSH2 (mutS (E. coli) homologue 2) are human homologues of an E. coli gene that encodes a protein involved in repair of mistakes in DNA replication.

Li–Fraumeni syndrome

Clinical features. Inheritance of only one functional copy of the p53 gene (see p. 123) predisposes to the development of several diverse tumours, usually in early adult life.

Disease-related gene. p53 (17p13.1) is a transcription factor that activates expression of a large number of genes which are thought to prevent accumulation of DNA mutations in cells.

Although germline mutations resulting in Li–Fraumeni syndrome are rare, mutations in p53 can be found in the many human malignancies, emphasizing the importance of this gene in protecting against the development of cancer.

Multiple endocrine neoplasia 1

Clinical features. A group of autosomal dominant disorders in which benign and malignant tumours arise in endocrine organs.

Disease-related gene. In multiple endocrine neoplasia 1 (MEN-1) defects occur in a gene encoding the menin protein (11q13). The function of menin is as yet unknown.

Neurofibromatosis type 1 (von Recklinghausen's disease)

Clinical features. An autosomal dominant disorder characterized by multiple pigmented skin lesions (café au lait spots and freckling in the axillae) and benign and malignant tumours, including neurofibromas and optic gliomas.

Disease-related gene. Neurofibromin (17q11) is thought to control cell proliferation by activating a Ras GTPase. Although DNA-based testing is available it is rarely used for prenatal testing or diagnosis. The exact function of neurofibromin is not yet fully understood.

Neurofibromatosis type 2

Clinical features. An autosomal dominant disorder characterized by bilateral benign tumours of the auditory nerves (acoustic neuromas). Other central and peripheral nervous tumours occur.

Disease-related gene. The neurofibromatosis 2 gene product has been named merlin, for moezin-ezrin-radixin like protein, because of its similarity to these cytoskeletal proteins. DNA-based mutation analysis is available clinically for the early detection of at-risk individuals (usually children of affected patients).

Retinoblastoma

Clinical features. Retinoblastoma is a malignant tumour of the retina affecting about 1 in 20 000 children. About 25% of cases are familial. Inherited cases of retinoblastoma usually present with the development of malignant tumours of the retina within the first 5 years. As more children survive following treatment with surgery or radiotherapy, it has become apparent that they are at increased risk of osteosarcoma and other tumours in later life.

Disease-related gene. The retinoblastoma 1 protein (13q14.2) is thought to act as a negative regulator of cell proliferation by sequestering a number of nuclear proteins involved in cell growth. Familial cases are dominantly inherited, so if a mutation is inherited on one chromosome, a sporadic mutation must occur on the other chromosome. Sporadic cases require that two separate mutations occur on both copies of chromosome 13.

Tuberous sclerosis
Clinical features. An autosomal dominant condition in which multiple benign tumours commonly occur in the skin, retina, brain and kidneys. Epilepsy and mental retardation are often associated.

Disease-related genes. The disease can be caused by mutations in either of two genes. *TSC1* (9q34) encodes the protein hamartin which has no clear homology to other vertebrate proteins. *TSC2* (16p13) encodes the protein tuberin which shows some homology to GTPase-activating proteins.

von Hippel–Lindau syndrome
Clinical features. An autosomal dominant condition characterized by the abnormal growth of capillary blood vessels to form angiomas. These often occur in the retina, the spinal cord and the cerebellum. Other tumours occur, including renal carcinoma and phaeochromocytoma in the adrenal gland.

Disease-related gene. The elongin-binding protein (3p26) is thought to regulate exit from the cell cycle.

Presymptomatic diagnosis is possible by DNA analysis, allowing surveillance for tumours in gene carriers.

Wilms' tumour
Clinical features. Wilms' tumour is an embryonal malignancy of the kidney that affects about 1 in 10 000 children.

Disease-related gene. One Wilms' tumour suppressor gene (*WT1*) has been located (11p13), and found to encode a transcription factor that

is critical to normal kidney and gonadal development. A second Wilms' tumour suppressor gene has been identified at 11p15, and linkage studies suggest that further loci may exist.

Cancer therapy

Cancer vaccines
Tumours often provoke an immune response against themselves, as evidenced by the detection of circulating tumour-reactive T lymphocytes, and the presence of tumour-infiltrating lymphocytes. However, tumours also protect themselves against immune reactions. For example, many tumours express only small amounts of MHC molecules, which are required to present tumour-derived peptides to the host's immune system.

A number of strategies are being developed to immunize patients against their cancers.

Immunization with tumour-specific peptides
Mutated oncogenes, such as p53, produce tumour-specific oncoproteins that can generate a cytotoxic T-lymphocyte response. Peptide fragments of such proteins could therefore be used as vaccines to immunize patients against their cancers.

One particular group of tumours lends itself particularly well to this form of therapy. B-cell lymphomas arise through the clonal proliferation of a single B cell. Each B-cell lymphoma therefore expresses a distinct antibody, with a unique variable region forming the antigen-binding site, on its surface (see p. 101). Advances in recombinant DNA technology make it possible to clone the variable region gene from lymphoma cells, and design a recombinant vaccine that fuses the variable region protein with other proteins such as GM-CSF (granulocyte–macrophage colony-stimulating factor) to make it more immunogenic.

Direct injection of a human leucocyte antigen gene not expressed by the tumour
The gene for a foreign human leucocyte antigen (HLA) is injected into the tumour in a form in which it can be taken up by the

tumour (e.g. as a DNA/liposomal complex; see p. 51). The hope is that in addition to recognizing the injected HLA as foreign, an immune response will be generated against other tumour antigens.

Gene therapy for cancer

Several approaches to gene therapy for cancer are currently being pursued.

• Retroviruses can be used to deliver specific therapy to tumour cells. For example, an enzyme involved in the activation of a cytotoxic drug can be linked to the promoter region of a gene that is preferentially expressed in the tumour.

• Tumour-infiltrating lymphocytes (obtained by biopsy of the tumour) can be infected with retroviruses containing human cytokine genes, such as tumour necrosis factor or interleukin 2. The lymphocytes are then reintroduced into the patient in an attempt to deliver high concentrations of cytokines to the tumour. An alternative approach is to transfect the cytokine gene into tumour cells, which are then reintroduced in the hope that cytokine secretion by the tumour cells will activate an immune response.

• Tumour suppressor genes or oncogenes could be manipulated within cancer cells. For example genes such as P53 could be introduced into cancer cells. Alternatively, retroviruses could be used to deliver antisense oligonucleotides (DNA sequences which bind to mRNA preventing its translation into protein; see p. 88), which interfere with the expression of mutant oncogenes.

Molecular classification of cancer

The identification of many genes involved in cancer may revolutionize the way in which tumours are classified. Pathologists have traditionally relied on histology to classify tumours. Classification according to genetic defects may improve prediction of clinical outcome and response to specific treatments. In addition, molecular assessment of tumour margins and regional lymph nodes may improve staging of tumours.

DNA MICROARRAYS

A DNA microarray is a slide or 'chip' which has been systematically dotted with DNA from thousands of genes that serve as probes for detecting which genes are active in different cell or tissues.

The use of DNA microarrays (see box above and p. 87) to simultaneously monitor expression of thousands of genes may allow a detailed study of the molecular basis of tumour growth.

Infectious diseases

Progress in molecular biology has relied on techniques used by viruses, yeast and bacteria to ensure their survival. These tools are now extensively used in the diagnosis and eradication of these microorganisms.

Diagnosis of infections

Polymerase chain reaction

The diagnosis of an infection usually requires culture, and identification, of the suspected infectious agent from samples obtained from the patient. Culture can be difficult or slow, resulting in inevitable delays in obtaining a diagnosis. This is particularly the case with certain bacteria (for example, tubercle bacilli and rickettsiae) and most viruses. PCR can be used to amplify DNA (or viral RNA) sequences which are specific for an infectious agent, allowing the rapid diagnosis of infections.

It is a useful tool in the diagnosis of viral infections, including hepatitis B and C, HIV and herpes simplex, and should prove of value in the diagnosis of bacterial infections such as tuberculous meningitis which can prove difficult to confirm using current bacteriological techniques.

Monoclonal antibodies

Monoclonal antibodies recognize target antigens with tremendous specificity and precision (see p. 101). This makes them ideal for detecting specific external antigens on microorganisms. Examples include *Legionella*, cytomegalovirus and herpesviruses.

Monoclonal antibody therapy in septic shock
Septic shock is a systemic response to infection which carries a high mortality despite advances in antimicrobial therapy and intensive care practice. Various inflammatory mediators, including the cytokine tumour necrosis factor and extracts of bacterial cell walls (endotoxins), have been identified as mediators of septic shock. This has prompted clinical trials of monoclonal antibodies which neutralize these agents. Although animal studies showed beneficial effects of these agents, results of clinical trials in patients have been less encouraging. Antibodies against tumour necrosis factor did not confer any survival benefit when used in human subjects with septic shock. Anti-endotoxin antibodies have been shown to be of benefit in a subset of patients with septic shock, but it may not be possible to predict which patients will benefit prospectively from therapy, and these agents have yet to enter routine clinical practice.

Vaccines and immunization

Vaccination against infectious diseases has been one of the greatest achievements of medicine, leading to the eradication of smallpox, and the control of viral infections (including poliomyelitis, mumps, measles and rubella) and bacterial infections (including whooping cough, tuberculosis, tetanus and diphtheria).

Vaccination involves the administration of either live infectious agents, which have been attenuated to render them harmless (e.g. the combined measles, mumps and rubella vaccines, vaccines against poliomyelitis and typhoid), or killed preparations derived from the plasma of infected individuals (e.g. the original hepatitis B vaccine) or culture of the microorganism (e.g. hepatitis A vaccine).

These preparations have potential disadvantages. Attenuated agents rarely cause disease, whereas preparing vaccines from infected plasma carries the risk of transmitting other infections. Furthermore it may prove difficult to culture the microorganism in sufficient quantities to make an inactivated product. Alternatively, it may be impossible to provide the necessary attenuation whilst retaining the ability to replicate without causing disease.

Recombinant proteins as vaccines
Recombinant DNA technology provides the opportunity to clone and express genes from infectious agents, and obtain recombinant protein products that can then be tested as vaccines. However, considerable difficulties have been encountered in expressing proteins in soluble forms which are immunogenic. This in part reflects the fact that the protein may be folded into a configuration which fails to induce the relevant immune response.

The only successful recombinant vaccine which has been produced to date is the hepatitis B vaccine. The surface protein of the hepatitis B virus, when expressed in yeast cells, forms particles which closely resemble the natural viral protein. These recombinant particles provoke a strong immune response against the hepatitis B virus.

Peptides as vaccines
The development of an immune response to an infection depends upon the agent containing molecules which are recognized as foreign. Substances which provoke immune responses are known as antigens. Antigens contain several sites or determinants, known as epitopes, which are capable of stimulating a protective immune response.

The simplest, and potentially safest, form of vaccine is therefore a peptide which is representative of an epitope present on the surface of the microorganism. With the availability of DNA sequencing techniques (see p. 77) the nucleic acid sequence of genes encoding potentially immunogenic proteins can be defined, and the amino acid sequence of peptides deduced. However, very few epitopes consist of linear amino acid sequences. Usually they are composed of discontinuous amino acid sequences that are brought together by folding of the protein. Identification of potentially immunogenic epitopes has therefore provided a major challenge.

Recombinant infectious vector vaccines

An alternative approach is to insert DNA from an infectious agent into an attenuated bacterial or viral vector. Following infection with the recombinant product, an immune response is generated against both the vector and the inserted gene product.

A variety of attenuated bacteria and viruses (including *Salmonella* and vaccinia, respectively) are currently under investigation as live vaccine vehicles.

DNA vaccines

The injection of plasmid DNA encoding antigens expressed by infectious agents can evoke strong and sustained humoral and cell-mediated responses. The plasmid DNA can be injected either directly or using a 'gene gun' that shoots tiny plasmid-coated beads into the body. The plasmid DNA is taken up by the recipient's cells, transcribed into RNA in the cell nucleus, and translated into protein that can act as an antigen. Although the vaccines cannot cause infection there is concern about integration of the DNA into the recipient's genomic DNA.

DNA vaccines are relatively easy to produce, and yield proteins that are expressed in their native state. Plasmid DNA is stable and does not require continuous cold storage, making the vaccines ideal for use in tropical areas. Trials of DNA vaccines for AIDS (see p. 131) and malaria are already under way.

Human immunodeficiency virus (HIV) infection

HIV-1 and HIV-2 are members of the lentivirus family of retroviruses. The virus preferentially infects CD4+ helper T lymphocytes leading to a decline in CD4 cell counts and impaired cell-mediated immunity. Eventually the immune system becomes clinically compromised and the patient develops the infectious, neurological and neoplastic complications characteristic of AIDS.

HIV-2 shares 45% sequence homology with HIV-1, and is found mainly in West Africa. It is less pathogenic *in vitro*, and transmission rates appear to be lower.

Viral transmission is either bloodborne from intravenous drug abuse or transfusion of blood or blood products, or through either homo- or heterosexual contact. Approximately 20% of children born to HIV-positive mothers are infected, some through breast feeding, which should be avoided.

The development of therapies for AIDS requires an understanding of how the HIV-1 virus integrates into the human genome, and how viral replication and viral gene expression are regulated.

The proviral genome of HIV-1 is 9–10 kb long, and has three main structural genes (Figs. 4.7 & 4.8).

• The *gag* (group-specific antigen) gene encodes the core protein antigens of the virion (intact virus particle). These are formed as the cleaved products of a larger precursor protein.

• The *pol* (polymerase) gene encodes the viral reverse transcriptase, and also the IN protein required for integration of viral DNA into the host genome.

• The *env* gene encodes the two envelope glycoproteins. These are synthesized in the form of the gp160 glycoprotein which is cleaved to generate gp120, the exterior envelope glycoprotein, and gp41, the transmembrane glycoprotein.

In addition a number of other genes encode protein products.

• The *pro* gene encodes the protease that cleaves the gag and pol protein precursors.

• The *vif* gene encodes a protein necessary for virion infectivity.

• The *nef* gene product functions as a negative factor for viral replication.

• The *tat* gene encodes a protein with trans-activating function. It interacts with the TAR (trans-activation response region) of the 5′-LTR (long terminal repeat), which contains regulatory sequences involved in viral gene expression.

• The *rev* gene encodes the regulator of virion protein, which determines whether structural

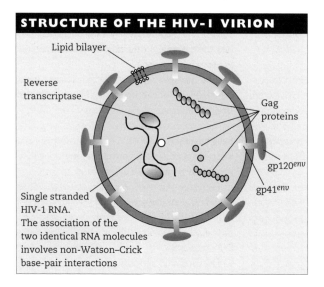

Fig. 4.7 The structure of the HIV-1 virion.

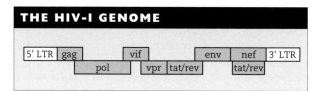

Fig. 4.8 Representation of the HIV-1 genome. The 5'- and 3'-LTRs (long terminal repeats) contain regulatory sequences. Several genes overlap.

genes are spliced from the viral mRNA, thereby determining whether only regulatory proteins or complete viral particles ready for nuclear export are made (Fig. 4.8).

When the HIV virion binds to a CD4 molecule on the cell surface a conformational change occurs in the envelope glycoprotein, and the virus enters the cell via fusion of lipid bilayers at the cell surface. The uncoated core of the virion then uses its viral reverse transcriptase to transcribe one of the two identical strands of positive-sense RNA into DNA. This DNA is duplicated by a host cell DNA polymerase, and migrates to the nucleus where it is integrated at a random site into the genome. Transcription of the integrated viral DNA is regulated by both host factors (such as the DNA-binding protein NFκB), and viral regulatory proteins such as the tat and rev proteins. Virally encoded proteins are processed and

assembled in the cytoplasm, and then bud from the cell surface as new infectious virions.

Therapy for AIDS

Inhibition of viral replication, using a combination of drugs to limit the emergence of resistance, is currently the mainstay of treatment. Zidovudine (azidothymidine, AZT), and the newer agents didanosine (ddI) and dideoxycytosine (ddC) are nucleoside analogues which bind preferentially to viral reverse transcriptase compared to human DNA polymerase. Although these drugs have led to a decline in AIDS incidence and mortality in developed countries, their use is limited by the cost, complexity and toxicity of current regimes. Furthermore, hopes that prolonged inhibition of viral replication may allow gradual eradication of the virus as infected cells die have proved unfounded. HIV-1 persists in latently infected cells and viral load rebounds if treatment is discontinued. Containment of the AIDS epidemic still requires the development of an effective vaccine, but the virus is ingenious in its ability to evade natural or induced immune recognition. HIV-1 keeps its weapons well hidden, and also mutates extremely rapidly during infection. This has important implications for the use of attenuated live viruses, which may mutate not only to escape immune recognition, but also to regain their pathogenic potential.

Targeting HIV entry into cells

Attachment of HIV-1 virions to target cells involves interaction of the gp120 glycoprotein with CD4, and members of the chemokine receptor family. CD4 binding induces a conformational change that helps expose the binding site for the chemokine receptor. The gp120 sequence contains five variable regions (V1 to V5), interspersed with conserved regions. The V3 loop may be particularly important in gp120-CD4–chemokine receptor interactions. Interaction of gp120 with the chemokine receptor induces a conformational change in gp120, which exposes a hydrophobic domain in gp41, initiating the fusion of viral and cell membranes.

The functional importance and exposed nature of gp120 appear to make it an ideal target for neutralization by antibodies, but here the virus displays its ingenuity in protecting itself. The highly conserved binding domains appear to be hidden within the structure of gp120, whereas the exposed regions are variable or masked by the addition of sugar moieties.

Live attenuated vaccines

High titre HIV-1 envelope-binding antibodies develop in infected individuals, but these often have poor neutralizing activity and do not limit viral replication. Stimulation of HIV-1-specific CD8+ cytotoxic T lymphocytes (CTLs) may be important, as CTLs appear to play a role in containing HIV-1 infection in infected individuals. It is unclear whether vaccination with attenuated viruses will be able to elicit the required immune response, and modified 'non-pathogenic' HIV viruses may be far from harmless. A naturally occurring nef-deleted HIV-1 eventually depleted CD4+ cells in humans, and a triple deleted simian immunodeficiency virus designed as a vaccine has caused AIDS in macaques.

Subunit vaccines

Recombinant HIV-1 envelope proteins are relatively inexpensive to produce, and considerable interest has been expressed in their use as subunit vaccines. In phase I/II clinical trials recombinant gp120 subunit vaccines failed to elicit neutralizing antibodies or specific CTL responses and did not protect against infection.

DNA vaccines

HIV DNA vaccines encoding envelope proteins can evoke neutralizing antibodies and CTL responses. They may provide ideal vaccines to elicit protective immunity, and are now in human trials.

Transplantation

Human leucocyte antigen (HLA) typing

Human leucocyte antigens are a family of glycoproteins that comprise the major histocompatibility complex (MHC) in humans and are encoded on the short arm of chromosome 6. There are three HLA class I molecules, known as HLA-A, HLA-B and HLA-C, that are expressed on the surface of all nucleated cells, and three HLA class II molecules, known as HLA-DR, HLA-DP and HLA-DQ, that are normally expressed on a much smaller subset of cells, particularly lymphocytes, although their expression on other cell types can be induced during immune reactions. The function of both classes of HLA molecules is to bind pieces of proteins (peptides) and display them on the cell surface where they can be recognized by circulating T lymphocytes. HLA class I molecules bind peptides derived from intracellular parasites, such as viruses, and present them to cytotoxic T cells, which kill virally infected cells. HLA class II molecules bind peptides derived from extracellular pathogens and present them to helper T cells, which help B lymphocytes to produce antibodies.

The genes encoding HLA antigens are extremely polymorphic, meaning that a large number of different alleles exist for each gene. Thus the pattern of HLA molecules expressed, known as the HLA type, varies considerably between individuals. Whilst this is probably important for the health of the population because of the broader resistance to pathogens, it makes organ transplantation much more difficult because the recipient mounts a strong immune response against any different HLA molecules expressed on the donor tissue. The extent to which the HLA type of the organ donor matches that of a potential recipient is an important determinant of the survival of the organ graft, and hence an important criterion for determining who receives an organ. Previous methods of HLA typing required days of culture or large panels of antisera, and involved complicated subsequent analysis. PCR provides a rapid method of HLA typing (known as tissue typing) prior to transplantation by testing different HLA-specific primers to see if they yield an amplification product.

Strategies for preventing organ rejection

T cells are the principal mediators of transplant rejection. In addition to engagement of the T-cell receptors by MHC molecules, T-cell activation requires an interaction between other cell surface proteins on the T cell and the cell presenting antigens in the context of MHC molecules (the antigen-presenting cell). These include CD28 and CD40 ligand on the T cell, and B7 and CD40 on the antigen-presenting cell. Once activated, T cells secrete soluble inflammatory mediators (cytokines) which then regulate the immune response.

The rejection process could be modified by transfer of genes that encode immunomodulatory cytokines to the transplant, or administra-

tion of recombinant proteins which interfere with T-cell activation. For example, survival of a transplanted mouse heart can be prolonged by retroviral-mediated transfer of the cytokine interleukin 10, which tends to suppress upregulation of HLA class II molecules. CTLA4Ig is a recombinant protein in which a homologue of CD28 is fused to part of an immunoglobulin molecule to create a soluble fusion protein that binds to the CD28 ligand B7.

Monoclonal antibody therapy in transplant rejection

Monoclonal antibodies against T-cell subsets have been extensively used to identify T cells in rejecting organs, and improve understanding of the rejection process. In addition many highly specific monoclonal antibodies against T-cell antigens have been developed as potential therapies for rejection. The most widely used has been the mouse monoclonal antibody OKT3 which recognizes CD3, which forms part of the human T-cell receptor. Many patients develop an antimouse antibody response which limits the use of this agent, but antibody engineering to 'humanize' OKT3 has been undertaken.

Xenotransplantation

Xenotransplantation is the transplantation of organs or cells between different species.

The severe shortage of donor organs has led to increasing interest in the use of animal organs for human transplantation. Although the immunological barriers to transplantation between species are formidable, the use of transgenic techniques (see p. 95) to express protective human genes in pigs has allowed limited survival of porcine organs transplanted into primates.

The transplantation of pig organs into primates results in hyperacute rejection, which occurs immediately after revascularization. It is mediated by binding of naturally occurring xenoreactive antibodies to graft endothelial cells, resulting in the activation of complement (see p. 101). The process is potentiated by the incompatibility of complement regulatory proteins in the transplant with the recipient's complement system—porcine regulators of complement activity do not limit human complement activation as effectively as their human counterparts.

Hyperacute rejection can be prevented by using transgenic donor pigs that express human complement regulatory proteins such as CD55 (decay accelerating factor; DAF), CD46 (membrane cofactor protein; MCP), and CD59 (an inhibitor of the complement–membrane–attack complex). These cell surface proteins act to downregulate complement activation (see p. 101).

If hyperacute rejection is overcome immunosuppression is required to prevent further immunological insults over the days and weeks which follow revascularization. These typically cause focal infarcts and haemorrhage, with or without cellular infiltrates.

Progress in the field has been sufficient for many countries to start regulating the practice, indicating that they consider the prospect of xenotransplantation as a reality. Concerns have been raised about the risk of transferring animal-borne pathogens to the recipient, and potentially to the public at large. Cross-species transmission of viral sequences has received considerable attention, and the potential for porcine endogenous retroviruses to integrate into the human genome is a particular concern.

One solution to the shortage of organs for transplantation may be the production of human tissues or organs by cloning. Like xenotransplantation, the prospect has become sufficiently real for a number of countries to introduce legislation concerning human cloning.

Cloning: from molecules to mammals—the birth of Dolly

Cloning (see p. 100) of mammals has now been achieved by nuclear transfer, in which a donor somatic cell is fused by electroporation (see p. 51) with a recipient enucleated oocyte. The first mammal to be cloned from a cell derived from adult tissue was Dolly the sheep. The nucleus of a cell from the mammary gland of a 6-year-old ewe was transferred to an enucleated unfertilized egg, and the reconstructed embryo transferred into a recipient ewe. Dolly proved to be a healthy lamb, and went on to display a sweater knitted from her wool in the British Science Museum.

Since Dolly's creation in 1995 successful cloning has been reported in cattle, mice, goats and, in September 2000, pigs.

Molecular biology is now of fundamental importance to laboratory science, commerce and clinical practice. Although motivated by potentially diverse interests, the ultimate goal is the development of new therapies that will benefit patients. The impact of molecular biology is now beginning to translate into such benefits.

Index

Page numbers in *italics* refer to figures and those in **bold** to tables.